613.25 DUF
Dufey, Chris, author.
Craving the truth : unlock the step-by-step
roadmap to rapidly drop "stubborn" fat, and
build the body of your dreams; ALL while
ditching traditional dieting forever.

Guelph Public Library

CRAVING
THE TRUTH

CRAVING THE TRUTH

Unlock The Step-By-Step Roadmap
To Rapidly Drop "Stubborn" Fat,
And Build The Body Of Your Dreams;
ALL While Ditching Traditional Dieting Forever

CHRIS DUFEY

613.25
DUF

Copyright © 2016 Chris Dufey
All rights reserved.

No part of this publication may be reproduced, stored in a retrieval system, or transmitted in any form or by any means, electronic, mechanical, photocopying, recording, scanning, or otherwise, except as permitted under Section 107 or 108 of the 1976 United States Copyright Act, without the prior written permission of the copyright owner.

Requests for authorization should be addressed to hello@chrisdufey.com.

Interior layout and design by www.writingnights.org
eBook formatted by www.writingnights.org
Book preparation by Chad Robertson

Readers should be aware that internet sites offered as citations and/or sources for further information may have changed or disappeared between the time this publication is made available, and when it is read.

Limit of Liability/Disclaimer of Warranty: While the publisher and author have used their best efforts in the publication of this work, neither author nor publisher makes any representations or warranties with respect to the accuracy or completeness of the contents of this work and specifically disclaim any implied warranties of merchantability of fitness for a particular purpose. No warranty may be created or extended by sales representatives or written sales materials. The advice and strategies contained herein may not be suitable for your situation. You should consult with a professional where appropriate. Neither the publisher, nor the author shall be liable for any loss of profit or any other commercial damages, including but not limited to special, incidental, consequential, or other damages.

DEDICATION

Lauren, Arlo, and Sunny.

Lauren, you're my best friend and wife that inspires me every day. Thank you for supporting me, believing in me, and being by my side as I follow my passion and can now share this with the world.

Arlo and Sunny, you are amazing and strong. I am blessed and am grateful every day that I get to be your father. Being able to play, laugh, cry, and soak in each moment with you is a blessing. All I want is for you to live the lives that has you following your passion and loving everything life has to offer.

CONTENTS

DEDICATION VII

CONTENTS IX

FOREWORD — THE PROMISE 1

ACKNOWLEDGEMENTS 5

INTRODUCTION 7

1 WHY YOU CAN'T LOSE THE WEIGHT 19

Ditch the Dieting and Get In the Best Shape of Your Life 23

2 WHAT IF EVERYTHING YOU'VE BEEN TOLD ABOUT DIETING … IS WRONG? .. 26

Calories Versus Hormones 34

3 IS YOUR DIET MAKING YOU FATTER? 35

4 "Calories Matter ... I Just Don't Count Them" 41

The Low-Calorie Trap and Damaging Your Metabolism 46
All calories are created equal: Lie 47
Why TEF Matters 50

5 Why Hormones Matter 53

6 Big 3 Hormonal Imbalances 60

The Blood Sugar Rollercoaster 60
The Stress Fat Factor 64
Is Your Brain Making You Fat? 69
How to Fix Your Gut Bacteria and Lose Weight 75

7 Why You Need to Sleep to Lose Weight 85

8 Why You Can't Copy My Diet 89

The Red Pill or The Blue Pill…? 96

9 The Truth to Losing Weight Fast and Keeping It Off Forever 97

10 "You Need to Eat Every 2-Hours to 'Stoke Your Metabolism.'" 103

11 "Breakfast is the Most Important Meal of the Day" 108

12 "You Should Eat Carbs at the Start of the Day" 111

13 "Eat Low Carbs to Lose the Weight." 114

14 "Cardio Is The Best Way To Lose Weight" 120

15 "Don't Worry About Supplements, They Are a Waste of Money" 124

16 Why Your Willpower is Failing You 130

17 The Truth of 'Detox' For Fat Loss 136

    The Magnificent 7 138
    How to Detox Your Body. 140

How to Detox Your Physical Body 143

18 THE 4 SIMPLE STEPS TO LOSING WEIGHT FAST..................................... 148

Eat Whole, Nutrient-Dense Foods 150
Move Every Day... 151
Bridge Your Nutrition Gap 152
Upgrade Your Lifestyle 152

19 THE MY BODY DIET 154

20 THE PVFC MEAL MODEL 158

The Quality of Your Food 163
Protein.. 164
Vegetables 165
Fats.. 166
Carbs 167
The Low Down on Fruit 169
"The Death of Fat Burning Foods" 170

21 ANSWERING: HOW MUCH DO I EAT? 172

22 CHOOSE YOUR EATING WINDOW . 182

16-8 188
The 24 Hour Fast 189

The Anti-Douche Guide to Intermittent Fasting 191
My Body Blends Intermittent Fasting for Fat-Loss Protocol: 194

23 MAKING EATING FOR FAT LOSS SIMPLE 196

The Best Ways to Get More Fiber 203
How Protein Can Help You Lose Weight 204

24 REFUEL MEALS AND THE DEATH OF CHEATING 209

How Your Brain Eats 214
The Real Benefits of a Refuel Meal Done Right
.... 220

25 WORKOUT LESS FOR FASTER RESULTS 226

26 METABOLIC RESISTANCE TRAINING 230

Metabolic Resistance Training 230

27 LESS RUNNING MORE MET CON CARDIO FOR FAT LOSS 235

How Often Should I Do This? 237
How Your Training Affects Your Hunger........239

14 THE YIN TO YOUR YANG YOUR WORKOUT PLAN 242

How Can Adrenal Problems Lead to Weight Gain? 246

29 INNER GAME - GOAL SETTING AND WILLPOWER.................................. 250

You Are the Placebo 252
Your Identity and Your Subconscious............255
Does This Sound Familiar..? 260
You Are Your Habits 262
Outcome Versus Behavior Focused. 269
What It All Starts With 270

30 LIFESTYLE.................................. 274

Sleep..275
The Wind Down Routine: 279
#1: Turn Off Your Electronics......................280
#2: Chill Out. 282
#3: Dark, Quiet and Cool. 283
Step 2: The Power of Your Chronotype. 283
Stress...286
Find a better way to deal with your stress......289
This Is How We Accelerate Your Fat Loss 290

31 5 STEPS TO BALANCING STRESS, ACCELERATING YOUR FAT LOSS AND FEELING LIKE "YOU" AGAIN 291

Start with the My Body Diet. 291
Mindfulness Practice - 2min of breathing to 20min of meditation 292
Do what you enjoy: 293
Movement: The Yin and the Yang 293
Sleep and Wind Down (just chill out more). .. 295
1. Switch off your electronics, phone, computer, and TV 296
2. Upgrade What You Eat and Drink Before Bed. 296
3. Prepare the 'Bat Cave.' 298

32 SUPPLEMENTS 300

The Truth to What Supplements WORK 300
Why We "Need" Nutritional Supplements 301
Why We Start with Quality over Quantity 308
The Foundation Stack 310
Fish Oil and Omega 3s 310
Fish Oil Enables You Lose Fat and Build Muscle. 311
Greens Superfood 313
Greens and Weight Loss 319
How Probiotics Can Help with Weight Loss .. 320
The Truth to Fiber Supplements for Weight Loss 323
How Protein Can Help You Lose Weight and Belly Fat 325

Why You Need to 'Test' Yourself 328

33 HOW TO GET IN THE BEST SHAPE OF YOUR LIFE 331

The 14-Day Metabolic Switch. 331
The 14-Day Jump Start Meal Plan 333
After the 14-Day Jump Start... 335
The 14-Day Metabolic Priming Phase 337
Quenching the Fire 342
Breaking the Habit of You 343
What's After the Metabolic Priming Phase?...349

34 THE ONE COMMON FACTOR TO MAKING YOUR MEAL PLAN EASY 351

The three Flavor Tender Meats: 356

35 THE KICKSTART WORKOUT GUIDE 359

Exercise order: 359
Tempo (speed of movement with each exercise): 360
Rest: 361
Intensity: 361
Workout 2 363

36 THE MY BODY DIET PROTOCOL ... 364

After The 14-Day Metabolic Switch 370

37 THE MY BODY FOR LIFE	374
REFERENCES	379
AUTHOR'S NOTE	390

FOREWORD
THE PROMISE

Are you frustrated from "trying all the diets," staying strict, working hard and still not being able to lose the weight…?

What if I could show you how to lose the unwanted weight, faster than you thought possible…?

What if I told you, you could have your dream body without having to press stop on your life, family, work, and responsibilities… WITHOUT having to starve yourself or battle daily craving…?

If that's what you want… then this book is for you.

You can wake up each morning and love the reflection in the mirror.

You can have the confidence that comes with being in the shape you want.

You can thrive each and every day by optimizing your brain and having vibrant health.

You can live your life not stressing over "what to eat," "when to eat," "how much to eat," "how to exercise," and the 101 questions that can plague us when we just want to be the best versions of ourselves.

The weight loss industry wants you to believe that it's hard, complicated, and that you need the 'radical weight loss diets,' pills and powders to ever have a chance of losing weight.

But you know that doesn't work.

And that's why it's time for a change.

In 4 weeks from right now, by following the simple guide I have for you here, you can dramatically transform your body, and more importantly, set yourself up for long-term success.

This book is written to get you in amazing shape. To burn fat off faster than you ever have before. But your full transformation does not end with these pages.

And I have to be brutally honest with you. This is always evolving. Even as I write these chapters I am constantly learning more, and tapping into the wisdom of the worlds best which grows what I can give you. This is why this book is just the beginning…

That's because the transformation you're looking for, where you're able to burn off the unwanted weight, feel confident in your body and have great health, continues with the free coaching guide I have set up for you.

Your Free Weight Loss and Body Transformation Guide is here:

http://cravingthetruth.com/bookbonus

This is where you get FREE access to the guide that includes:

- The exact starting meal plan that includes the Metabolic Priming Phase.
- Shopping list and grocery guide so you can start straight away.
- The recipes that are our favorites and shows you how to quickly make the meals you look forward to without the fuss.
- The workout program for gym or home that matches your starting meal plan.
- The step-by-step coaching guides that include the videos I've personally recorded that are matched with your body so that you have a more tailored plan to suit you.
- Access to the My Body Blends community for all the live streams, guides, me and the team helping you along. As well as joining the like-minded people that create the support you can't get anywhere else.

Start with our famous Kickstart guide plus access into the bonus section to get the specials worth over $250 by going to:

http://cravingthetruth.com/bookbonus

ACKNOWLEDGEMENTS

I want to deeply thank everyone that has been a part of this book coming to reality. These people below have had a profound impact on me. THANK YOU for being world-class and delivering huge value to us all.

Mary Shenouda	Brad Schoenfeld	Reed Davis
Tim Ferriss	Dr. John Beradi	Jason Swannick
John Romaniello	Craig Ballytine	Jay Ferrugia
Marc David	Scott Stevenson	Bob Rokoawski
Mike Nelson	Ryan Munsey	Jade Teta
Jonathan Bailor	Kamal Patel	Barry Sears
Shelby Starnes	Damon Haymow	John Meadows
Ted Ryce	Ben Coomber	Phil Graham
Vince Del Monte	Nick Tumminello	Tyler Tolman
Mark Buckley	Derek Sivers	Dr. Mark Hyman
Robb Wolf	Dave Asprey	Dr Steve Gundry
Chris Kresser	Ben Pakulski	James Altucher
Rob Hanly	Robert Sapolsky	Dr. Robert Lustig
Dr. Barry Sears	Katrina Ruth	Dr. Vera Tarman
Robb Wolf	Chris Kresser	Charles Duhigg's
Dr Bryan Walsh	Dr. Steve Gundry	Christian Maurice

Vince Del Monte   Charles Poliquin   John Kiefer

Mike T Nelson   Dr. Joel Fuhrman,   Tyler Tolman

Dr. Michael Eades   Steven Witherly   Nick Tumminello

Dr. Hendricks Gay.   Ann Gabryiel   Jesse Elder

Ben Pakulski   Dr. Michael Breus   Dr. Joe Dispensa

Damon Haymow   Ted Ryce

INTRODUCTION

"If it were just more information we need. We would all be billionaires with perfect abs."

- DEREK SIVERS

One of the biggest problems you face is that you are overloaded with information.

If you're anything like my clients, you're busy. And you've "tried all the diets" but are still confused about how to get in shape.

You've counted the calories, cut the carbs, done the detox's, drank the shakes, sweated through the endless workouts. But when you look in the mirror, you're not happy with what you see.

You've read their articles.

You've watched their videos.

You've listened to their podcasts.

But the truth is the endless amount of information that can have you feeling so overwhelmed - is not working for you.

The mainstream and 'guru' advice is not working for you, points the finger back at you, and is telling you that you just need to work harder and have more self-discipline.

This book is the answer to how to get in the best shape of your life.

If you're like me, you've probably asked yourself "why is a smart person like me, stuck with such a simple problem of losing weight?"

And the truth is; It's not your fault.

The traditional diets are setting you up for failure. You will have to battle through the three major problems of dieting each time, which are hunger, cravings, and low energy.

95% of people fail to lose weight and keep it off, with many actually gaining more weight than when they began the diet. And now, science is showing that this yo-yo dieting is actually making it harder for you to lose weight after every effort.

Dieting is actually making you fatter!

So much for the old, traditional weight loss advice, and well-educated nutritionists who are well versed in prescribing a 'diet.' But it's the compliance, it's the ability for you to follow it whilst living life, and sticking with these important habits of success that is missing.

Diets have failed both you and me, and that's why I want to walk you tough what's going to switch on your fat burning at a cellular level. And more importantly, have you living with vibrant health and happily getting on with your life.

I'm not the guru standing on the stage giving you another "top 5 tips for weight loss." This book is written for you because I was exactly where you are at right now.

This all started with my own journey of trying all the diets, depriving myself. Thinking I was just destined to always be overweight and unhappy. It's a dark hole that I know so many others feel trapped in. And this is why I felt the urge to write this for you.

I was a heavily overweight kid and teenager. My weight held me back from doing the things that I wanted to and stopped me from enjoying the simple pleasures of life because I was so caught up with how insecure I felt about my body.

This will give you the answers to "what do I eat?" and "how much do I eat?" Along with what your training and exercise should really be, what nutrients and supplements your body needs.

But more importantly, this reveals the easy to use advice that the world's top experts use for you to transform your body and life.

This book is the bringing together the behind the scenes look into the secrets the world top experts use. I'm giving you a backstage pass to having the advice from the best of the best.

Importantly, this is also NOT going to have you counting calories, doing tedious workouts, or depriving yourself of your favorite foods.

And that's why I want to introduce you to Chaz and Nicola in just a second.

Most of my clients and members come to me because they are fed up, they say they've "tried all the diets," and nothing works. They feel like giving up on ever 'being in shape' but want to give it one more go, as deep down, they truly want to have the confidence, feelings, and emotions for when they lose the weight.

At first, when they see the plan I have for them, they think I'm crazy. Everything they have read on the internet, in books, and learned about weight loss is the opposite of what I'm giving them. When I walk them through the reasoning for why (which I will do in the following chapters), they are happy to give it a go.

To their amazement, their body starts to change, and they see and feel the difference within the first few weeks. Then, they continue to get leaner and are usually in shock as it's all happening while not going through the hunger and cravings that they've battled through before.

For over 12 years now, I've been coaching body transformations around the world. My clients have ranged from mum and dads, CEO's, politicians, top bikini and fitness models, actors, and even Arab Sheiks.

Now, I get to write this book while sitting in my home office in Bali where I live with my wife and two daughters.

This book is for the 'every day' real person. So much of the wrong and regurgitated fat-loss advice is being perpetuated from trainers who are only telling you what to do because that's what works for them.

I've been a fitness model before and competed around the world. And the truth is, there is a big difference between what you need to do to get in peak condition to step in front of cameras and on a stage in the leanest physique possible, compared to being lean, strong, and happy in everyday life.

Let me introduce you to Chaz.

Chaz came to me wanting a change and in total confusion of what to do. After spending years focusing on his career, he found himself out of shape. One thing that I love about Chaz is that he committed to turning it all around and just needed to know how.

After just the first 4 weeks, he had lost 7.5 kilos. The most dramatic change was that he had clearly gained muscle at the same time, as his physique had totally transformed. Best of all, it was super simple for him to follow each day. He could happily get on with each day while having more than enough time for his training and loving the meals he got to eat.

This is where most diets have failed. They get you to focus on the wrong thing, and often, it's easy to fall prey to the 'eat less and exercise more' advice.' This only has you seeing food as the enemy, and you trying to stick with low-calorie diets.

This is why I also want to introduce you to Nicola.

Nicola was determined and on a mission. The only problem was that she was staying strictly to diets, training hard, and often exercising most days. And still not being able to lose the weight. Especially, the stubborn fat, which is where you have those parts of your body that are hard to lose no matter how much overall weight you lose.

Being very busy and often traveling with work, the diets she was trying to follow before she came to me were often very difficult to stick to. From what foods she was allowed, to when she could eat, and how many times she could eat.

Her transformation using the methods I will show you is a great example of how to dramatically transform your body. Especially from the 'hard to lose' areas. We had her eating more food, less time in the gym, more time with family and getting greater results.

I know how to do this because my specialty is NOT working

with high-end athletes. It's transforming the bodies of busy, everyday men and women who need quick results. Without it being confusing or time-consuming.

My days are full, being a dad of two daughters and running two businesses, and I still want to be able to have time and energy to be a great husband, have a social life, and look after myself.

This means that I had to find a better way.

The rulers of the health and fitness industry don't want you to know:

You don't need to repeatedly be trying crash diets in an effort to look good for the beach, a special occasion, or just to feel confident with your reflection.

You can save yourself $100's to $1000's each year by not falling prey to the over-hyped supplements and products that don't work.

The biggest problem you face is continuing to try the diets and plans that haven't worked for you. We've all seen the people that are in the gym day in, day out for years and who have never changed body shape, but they are still chasing the results they want.

This is NOT a one size fits all plan. The science applies to everyone, though the exact recipe you need to follow is individual to you. You will see why trying to follow a 'cookie-cutter' diet in the coming pages will not work for you. This is where I want to be by your side helping you. So that you can easily use the guiding principles I'm about to show you, and happily get on with your life.

So many people are trying to force feed you one diet to follow. But there is no perfect diet. What works for you now might not work for you in a year from now. And the people constantly searching for "the perfect diet" are asking the wrong question.

The right question is, "what is right for you, now?"

The more failed dieting efforts, and the older you get, the harder it can be.

But first, I have to be honest with you.

This is where this book is NOT about weight loss. It's really about fat loss. And the two are very different. Just losing weight and having the scales tell you that you're lighter is a false promise.

That's why, if you want to be free from what the scales say and you want to burn off body fat, so you look, feel, and function the way you want each day, then this book is for you.

This is where the difference between information and transformation live.

It's the caterpillar that turns into a butterfly. It's the unhappy, frustrated, and overweight person that turns into a lively, positively impacting human who suddenly has the energy and confidence to achieve their dreams. And seeing these transformations not only with just people's bodies, but their lives and how they go through their lives is one of the best things about what I do.

Yes, this book is about transforming your body.

Having you lose the weight and build the body you want. But it goes a lot deeper than that. I know that when you do it the right way, you can have your body transformation be the starting block that opens up to a happier, healthier you.

You being the best version of yourself.

Peter Sage so powerfully says, "to know and not to do, is not to know." And I work on using this in every part of my life. How many people do you know (you could be one of them) who know all the facts and figures about diet and nutrition, yet fail to lose the weight? You know that you shouldn't be eating a certain way, yet you keep falling off the wagon.

And to throw in another quote from someone a lot smarter than me, Albert Einstein said, "nothing happens, until something moves." This talks directly to you, your body, and your life. Transformation happens because you DO something.

The simple act of taking information you've learned and applying that information in the real world is the difference between where you are and where you want to be. And by creating the habits and behaviors, so you are then doing the right actions on autopilot, you will be taking the steps toward what you want to achieve.

This is why I'm excited that you are reading this right now.

I wrote this book for you to create your own transformation. As from my own personal experience and with coaching people for over 12 years around the world, I'm happy that the ego of us wanting to look better, be more attractive, and feel sexy is a great starting position.

The real truth is that I know that by feeding your body the right foods, by changing the daily actions you take, and having the habits and behaviors that make it 'effortless' and automatic for your body to burn off the unwanted fat, your mitochondria, the ancient bacteria that are now living in each of our cells that produce the basic building blocks of energy in our bodies will be more effective and efficient. Your brain will be functioning better, giving you better clarity of thought and mental power.

You won't be on a rollercoaster of ups and downs with your moods, emotions, or energy throughout the day.

You won't be feeling "off" and just not your normal self from feeding yourself the wrong foods.

You will be taking care of your health. As this is about putting the 'health' back into the health and fitness world. Because in the desperate attempt to lose weight, the mainstream media has latched onto the fact that they can spew lies and sell incredible amounts of products that not only don't work, can actually cause harm.

You'll feel empowered from knowing how to easily go through each day truly taking care of your body and your brain.

And simply being able to get on with your life to enjoy it. Not constantly battling with hunger, cravings, or worrying about how you look.

This life is far too short and way too amazing to be bogged down with weight loss problems.

And that's why I want you to discover that you have the power.

Far too many people think they have lost control.

That their genetics means they are meant to be overweight. Or, they just don't have the willpower to follow a diet to lose weight. Or the power to say no to the foods they know they shouldn't be eating so often.

And this is where I have to say -

NO!

You never lost control.

This isn't about you "taking back control." Because you never lost it.

When you take responsibility, you're not a victim, and when you're not a victim, you can do something about it.

That's why this book is NOT the holy grail answer and silver bullet. This is a guide that shows you how to find what is best going to work for you, your body, and your lifestyle.

No one single piece of paper that is a "diet" is going to best work for you. And you're going to discover in the coming chapters just how easy it can be for you go through each day nourishing your body, performing at high levels, and getting into the best shape of your life.

And that's the starting step to not just changing your body, but changing your life.

CRAVING THE TRUTH

Unlock The Step-By-Step Roadmap
To Rapidly Drop "Stubborn" Fat,
And Build The Body Of Your Dreams;
ALL While Ditching Traditional Dieting Forever

CHRIS DUFEY

1
WHY YOU CAN'T LOSE THE WEIGHT

Dieting is making you fat…

As I've always laughed when people have said to me "Oh, it's easy for you, you've got great genetics."

Let me tell you how I've really come to be writing this for you right now.

As a kid and a teenager, I was obese.

The getting picked on at school. The teasing. The lack of confidence to not only approach girls, but just to be happy - to smile - was a daily struggle.

Finally, the shame became too much. I had to do something about it, and it started with mustering up the courage to join a gym.

This quickly moved onto reading everything possible on training, diets, and supplementation.

But, frustration quickly set in as seeing any results was slow.

And all the articles, books and advice were confusing to me and conflicting each other. One article tells you to cut all carbs out and follow an Atkins or Keto Diet. Another says you should be eating more carbs.

Finally, after literally traveling the world, seeing the best coaches, sitting in the seminars, and spending countless hours training and coaching clients to lose weight, I cracked the code.

At least I thought so at the time…

I competed as a fitness model around the world and was able to get my clients into incredible shape. But there was something seriously wrong.

The all-consuming goal of "being in shape" had started to eat away at my relationships, happiness, and life. The constant thinking and worries about sticking exactly to the diet and training plan were becoming ridiculous.

Carrying around Tupperware's of food to make sure I was eating the right foods at the right time. Prioritizing my training over everything else.

And then it hit me.

"This has to be so simpler."

This was not the man, husband, and father I wanted to be.

For me now writing this for you, it's knowing that you can be the person you want to be. You can have it all.

You will lose weight easily and stay in shape all year round. Not having to battle with hunger or cravings.

You will be able to live a life. Go out with friends, and be social without having to stress over every morsel of food you put in your mouth.

You will have the energy to thrive; from waking up to going to bed. Never dragging yourself through the days with low energy.

You will be the best version of yourself.

As when I finally cracked the code to losing weight, being in great health and piecing together the key principles that work, I became known as the "trouble-shooter for weight loss." To get clients into shape, when they hadn't been able to do it themselves.

But, before I show you how the typical "eat less and move more" approach to weight loss is making you fatter and making it harder for you to lose the weight, I want to share this drastic truth with you.

After a grueling football game, where each of the players is battered and bruised, with so much at stake and so much effort and hard work put into trying to win the game, the head coach of the losing team walks into the crowded media pit to answer the questions.

With the lights and camera squarely pointing on him, he's asked with direct force, "why did you lose?"

After clearing his throat and thinking hard about the question, he answers…

"We scored too few points, and the other team scored too many points."

Now, let's bring this stark truth into the light with how this answer is just as crazy as why millions of people - and this could be you (likely so, because you are reading this) - are struggling with losing weight.

The mainstream advice you're told to solve your weight problems is, "eat less food, and move more." Basically, pointing the finger at you, and saying that you are a lazy glutton, and that's why you're not losing weight.

Now the answer the coach gave above is entirely accurate. BUT, it is not the cause of why the team lost. It's just the definition of what happened. That's why, when someone tells you to lose weight by eating less and moving more, it's NOT helpful.

There is clearly a deeper cause that is creating the problem, and that is why I have written this book for you. Over the coming chapter, I'm going to show you why it's happening, and then importantly, as a coach, I'm going to guide you through the 'how to lose the weight and have a huge domino effect' that will positively improve your life. This will include being more confident, having more sex, and having a better quality of life.

Kamal Patel is a nutrition researcher with an MPH and MBA from Johns Hopkins University and is on hiatus from a Ph.D. in nutrition in which he researched the link between diet and chronic pain. It's the fantastic work that he, along with the team at examine.com do that brings to light what the science says with supplementation and nutrition. The beauty of examine.com is they are the unbiased source for supplements and nutrition. They have spent tens of thousands of hours collating the latest scientific research.

Which is why I recommend them as a resource for you to use to keep yourself updated. And why I use Kamel, examine.com, and the many other experts and leaders that you are going to be introduced to through the pages to come.

Ditch the Dieting and Get In the Best Shape of Your Life

Every time you start a diet and follow the mainstream 'eat less and move more' advice, it's damaging your metabolism. And this damage is making it harder for you to lose weight and making your stubborn hard to lose spots even more stubborn.

Your body is made to adapt to the environment it's in. And your body goes through 'adaptive thermogenesis' (or a simpler term that I'll use going forward with you 'metabolic slowdown'), which is a slowing down of your metabolism to match the lowered food (calorie) intake and an increase in energy expenditure.

This, in turn, creates an unbalanced metabolism when you try to continue to follow the traditional weight loss diets.

YES! We need a calorie deficit to be able to burn body fat and lose weight, but we also need proper hormonal balance. This is where the 'eat less, move more' weight loss advice fails, as it only takes care of a part of the solution. It lowers your calories in some way or another.

This is where you create a hormonal and metabolic storm that makes fat loss harder and can lead to health issues. As key metabolic hormones, such as leptin and ghrelin (which tie in with your hunger), and thyroid (which is to do with your metabolism) cause the common problems with increased hunger and cravings, low daily energy, and a slowed metabolic rate.

This is why these styles of diets set you up for long-term failure.

In the short term, absolutely, you will lose weight, especially, scale weight, but it's not setting you up for long-term success. The short-term results are then outweighed soon after, as you can easily gain back the weight you lost and possibly gain even more. And, it will be even more stubborn for you to lose.

"Weight Loss Resistance" is what I'm here to reverse for you with this book. Just like the many clients that have come to see me, they've all followed the traditional diets, and they didn't work for them.

Unfortunately, your body doesn't care about getting lean, so you feel sexy, attractive, and confident. It's worrying about staying alive, and when your body perceives the stress of famine and starvation, it's going to make changes that keep you alive for longer during a famine.

These changes will be biochemical and hormonal, things that increase hunger and cravings so that you go on the hunt for food. The reason why you feel lethargic and have low energy is because your body is trying to get you to slow down, move less, and conserve energy. This can also be coupled with the problem that on a cellular level, your mitochondria aren't able to produce energy as efficiently as before, due to malnutrition.

A common scenario can look like this: A new client has been dieting and trying to lose weight for many months, even years, and is totally stuck. They've continued to cut back their calories, cut down their carbs, and increase their exercise. And step-by-step, they are now following a low-calorie diet with 1-2 hours of training per day, and they are still not getting leaner.

They have spent thousands of dollars on supplements, especially focusing on the more potent 'fat burners,' which are just over-stimulating their nervous system.

The concoction of stress builds in their body with:

- The daily stress, we all have to a degree, with living a modern life of being busy and having a host of responsibilities.
- The nutritional stress of under-eating for a prolonged time, especially cutting back or out certain foods and macronutrients.
- The mental stress and constant worrying of not being in the body shape they want, and why they aren't able to lose weight.
- An over-stimulated nervous system from the 'fat burner' supplements and stimulants, such as caffeine.
- The physical stress of high amounts of training, usually coupled with a low focus on recovery.

What we commonly see is tired, hungry, frustrated, and confused men and women who are fed up with not being able to lose weight and get in shape.

But over the next chapters, I'm going to show you why it's not your fault.

You've been given the wrong, misleading information. And what you need to be able to get the body and health you want, is so much simpler.

2
WHAT IF EVERYTHING YOU'VE BEEN TOLD ABOUT DIETING … IS WRONG?

When it comes to you answering the many questions that flood your head when you want to lose the weight and 'get into the best shape of your life.' The enormous amount of information when it comes to diet, exercise, supplements, and lifestyle habits have a common theme.

And it reminds me of the 'study' that was done on monkeys…

A group of scientists put a bunch of monkeys into an enclosure. Though this enclosure was slightly different from a normal habitat that monkeys would live in. They added a ladder, a bunch of bananas at the top of the ladder and had water sprinklers all over the roof.

When they let the monkeys lose into their new enclosure, it didn't take long for them to find out that there were bananas at the top of the ladder. And so, one monkey gets hungry and starts heading up the ladder. Before the monkey could get the top of the ladder, the scientists turn on the cold-water sprinklers, and all the monkeys get hosed and consequentially go nuts.

After a few more times of trying to climb the ladder to collect the prize of the bananas, the monkeys figured out that it wasn't a good idea. The bananas at the top weren't worth the effort if they all kept getting drenched in ice cold water.

Then the scientist did something interesting. They replaced one of the monkeys, with a new monkey. And this new monkey goes strolling on into the enclosure and soon see's the bananas at the top of the ladder. So he runs on over and starts heading up the ladder. It didn't take long before all the other monkeys pounced on him and beat him back down. He was taught the lesson to not head up the ladder, or you'll get your ass handed to you and beat down.

The scientists kept replacing one old monkey with a new one, and the same behavior kept happening. The monkey would want to head up the ladder, and the rest kept beating them back down. Then all the original monkeys were replaced with new monkeys that had never been soaked in the icy cold water. And whenever a monkey wanted to head up, they were beaten back down.

This is how much of the fitness industry is the same. Because if you were to ask all the new monkeys, why do you not let anyone go up the ladder? They would answer "because that's what we've always done."

And this is exactly what's going on with much of the fitness industry. The same perpetuating lies are being regurgitated over and over again. And just like Tony Robbins says, "the quality of your life is up to the quality of your questions." For me personally, I was stuck in a fat body and depressed with working so hard and 'doing everything right,' yet still not being able to lose weight. It took me asking different questions, and to look behind the curtain as to what different methods caused what outcomes and to understand the 'why.'

So, it's easy to have the foundational principles in place, and then be able to tailor what's needed for you to wash away the confusion and frustration from wasted time and effort.

This easy factor is one of the most important aspects of what is going to work for you. Because if you find it too hard to follow a program, and you can't stick with it, then it's never going to get you the long-term results you want.

This is why I want to introduce you two very special people in my life.

Especially for when it comes to the fact that you can completely turn your life around, and in the way James Altucher puts so well. You can 'choose yourself.'

One of the biggest complaints I hear is that the diets and weight loss programs that have failed so many, forced you to lose your social life so you can stick to it. And if you're like me (and the entire My Body Blends community), you want to be able to spend time with friends and family and not feel like you're missing out on life because your diet is so restrictive.

The two people I want to introduce you to are Suzanne and Glenn. My wife's mother and father-in-law, for which I am blessed to have as a part of my family. This is close to me because when we really boil down what we are talking about here, it's that we want ourselves, our loved ones, and our community to be in the best health both physically and mentally.

For me, this includes having Suzanne and Glenn living long and prosperous lives. So when they asked me to help them turn things around with their weight and health, I jumped at the opportunity. And we can let the photos speak for themselves. In just a matter of a few months, they have dramatically re-shaped their bodies and improved their health.

All by following a plan that was very basic and simple. And that's by design. Because, by having the easy to follow plan, Suzanne, Glenn, myself, and you can stick with it for the long-term. And this doesn't mean that you can't have fast results. Because you most certainly can and will by following the My Body Diet.

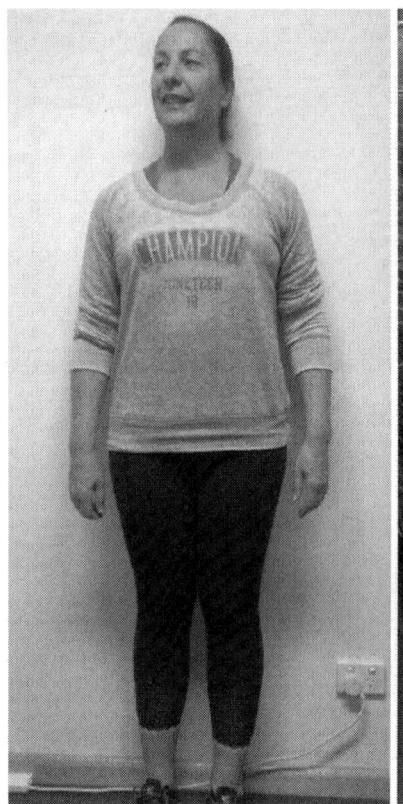

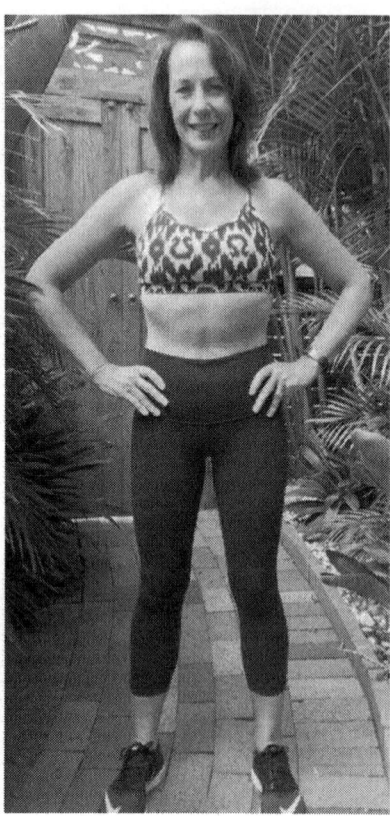

Here is what Suzanne has to say about it…

"We were both in a bad habit of eating way too many carbohydrate-heavy foods, drinking too much alcohol, and doing the same exercise over and over.

Chris' program re-educated us on what we should be eating. And we didn't completely give up alcohol. Being on a program like this also gives more structure and variety to your training and makes you accountable. Chris give us an easy to read and follow program - which is, in fact, our new way of life" - Suzanne McDougall.

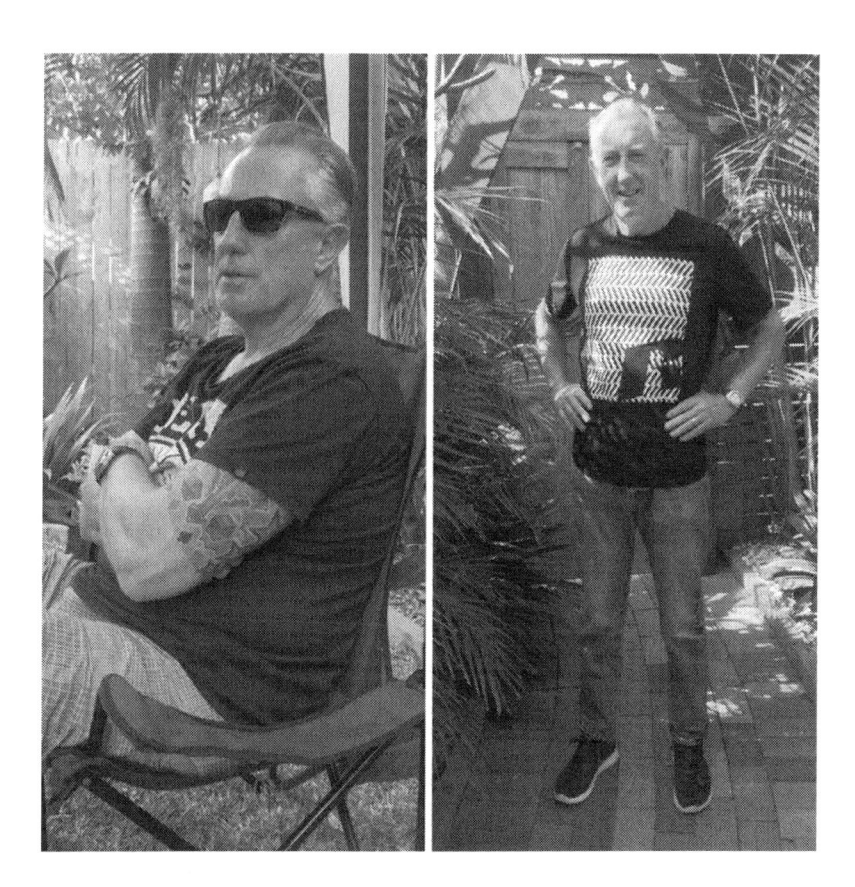

Now, another one of the biggest problems that can be holding you back from getting in shape is your bias.

> "Entertain the thought without embracing it"
>
> - Aristotle.

Talking diets and what foods we should be eating can be as touchy as religion and politics.

It was the unconscious biases I had believed in for so many years that held me back and stopped me from getting the results I wanted.

And it can be the very same for you right now.

One of the most powerful forces of the human psyche is to stay congruent with the ideas it carries with itself. This is why we can find it so hard to make a change, as our ego then has to admit it's wrong. But this is absolutely necessary for progress in all areas of our life.

For this book to be a life changer, and I know it can be for you (I'm slightly biased), you need to let go of your current beliefs about dieting. Many people still try to hold onto things that don't work. And this is why I'm going to show you why on so many levels; that millions of people are failing to burn off unwanted body fat and get into shape.

This also means we need to redefine 'diet.' As I don't want the word diet, to be associated with low calories, deprivation, hunger, and the like. This is why I want you to embrace the My Body Diet, and see that the only real way you can take back control, get in shape, and happily get on with your life is understanding that you are an individual and that your nutrition, movement, and lifestyle need to be set up to suit you.

Rob Hanly is someone that I've thankfully been able to learn much from for the past few years. And when Rob talks, you listen. It was when Rob shared with me a basic formula for how he was looking at how we were dealing with life. And I want to share this with you now, as it ties in perfectly with how we upgrade your lifestyle for long-term results.

Here is how he 'leverages the feedback loops to eliminate emotionalism.'

What I do > How I feel.

And as he says, "If the arrow flips, my output suffers and quantity and quality," Because what you do is more important than how you feel. After all, as a former SAS operator has been quoted as saying…

> "Since when did I need to feel like doing something in order to do it."

The My Body Diet approach understands that you are a unique person who can have amazing results using the guiding principles that I'll show you very soon, but then, taking it one step further, and tailoring each decision moving forward to suit you without any confusion.

It's blending together the proven methods with the right recipe that suits your body and your lifestyle. This isn't a cookie-cutter plan like the others you have followed, it teaches you how to win against weight loss resistance and see fast results while setting yourself up for long-term success.

This is where you need to let go of your bias of what nutritional regimes or beliefs you have. You can approach this in a very new way now by using this book, letting go of all everything that hasn't worked for you, and that includes the excessive workouts and calorie counting.

The difference for you now is going to be profound by moving from the method that focuses on just weight loss by counting calories to true fat loss, which brings about the hormonal balance and metabolism for long-lasting results.

Calories Versus Hormones

- The importance of both
- The body doesn't work
- The role of insulin
- How hormones relate to fat loss

If losing the unwanted weight and getting in shape was as easy as just eating fewer calories than you burn, then we would all have a 6-pack.

The truth is, our bodies don't act like a calculator. And why many gurus and most trainers have it wrong is because they are only focusing on part of the problem, which is why I'm going to walk you through the importance of your hormones, and the simple steps you can take to start to balance these.

The other problem is you're a human. Full of emotions, feelings, and living a real life, which means it can be stressful; responsibilities and things can get in the way, which means you can't follow a 1-page perfect diet for the rest of your life.

On top of this, your body is always changing. This is why you can't just have one diet, or meal plan, for the rest of your life. This is why I'm here to give the power back to you, so you can make smart decisions for the rest of your life rather than depending on a diet. This is also why I want to show you the guiding principles and get you started on the best plan possible.

3
IS YOUR DIET MAKING YOU FATTER?

Could the weight loss diets you've been following before actually be making you fatter, and harder for you to lose weight?

YES!

You're about to find out why eating less does not cause fat loss.

And to show how the mainstream advice for weight loss is flawed, we can look at the quote from George Bray from the Pennington Biomedical Research Center; "*The reduction of energy intake continues to be the basis of…weight reduction programs… [The results] are known to be poor and not long-lasting.*"

> **Bec Hoc**
> September 16 at 2:42pm · Melbourne, Australia
>
> At this rate I'll be in my jeans by... Summer lol! Ever wish you made a call earlier? 💕💕 #programworks

> **Lee Duncan**
> May 27 at 4:08pm
>
> Hey Chris Dufey, this stuff works! I've recorded food and weight each day in Myfitnesspal - dropped over 4lbs since Monday morning. That's despite going out for a curry on Thursday night (no rice, naan or booze) and a bottle of Cava with our Friday night supper. I'm grateful to you buddy. Looking forward to shifting a few more this next week. Have an awesome weekend.

This is going to ruffle some feathers, but you're going to see right now how I'll walk you through three of the main hormonal imbalances, that when you try to lose weight the wrong way, actually make you fatter.

What usually happens (not anymore after you read this book) when you follow a traditional diet, you drop your calories, eat less food, and ramp up your exercise. Our bodies are adaptive organisms, and we want to find and stay in homeostasis. So your body is essentially going to fight back against the changes you are making.

This is why we can see the more times you diet, the harder it is for you to lose weight. Because you are going to go through 'metabolic adaptations.' These adaptations will give you:

- Reduced energy expenditure and slow metabolic rate

through reduced NEAT (Non-Exercise Activity Thermogenesis).
- Lowered thyroid hormone; another reason why you have a lower energy expenditure.
- Reduction in sympathetic nervous system activity.
- Reduction in resting and exercise energy expenditure.
- Increased mitochondrial efficiency, so that your body can run on less fuel.
- Increased insulin sensitivity – This is a good thing when it's muscle that has increased insulin sensitivity. But this is increased sensitivity of fat cells. Meaning that your fat cells are better able to suck in nutrients and be stored as fat.
- Increased hunger hormones, such as Ghrelin.
- And you will see the three major hormonal imbalances, and how they work together to make it harder for you to lose weight.

These metabolic adaptations or metabolic slowdowns create an 'energy gap' that is the reduction of how much your energy burns throughout each day to bridge the gap left from the lowered amount of food you are eating. It also wants to make you eat more food as a secondary way to close this gap.

The University of Geneva researchers discovered in a study that the "Eat Less Group" metabolisms were burning body fat over 500% less efficiently and had slowed down by 15% by the end of the study. They remarked: "These investigations provide direct evidence for the existence of a specific metabolic component that contributes to an

<u>elevated efficiency of energy utilization during refeeding after low food consumption,</u>" or once eating less stops.

So your body is craving more food, with your brain actively signaling you to eat more by largely increasing your hunger hormone ghrelin.

Then we have your body slowing its metabolic rate with 'adaptive thermogenesis.'

Another issue that comes with the metabolic adaptations with failed diets is the changes in your body fat set point. As it's the number of fat cells you have that mainly dictates the amount of fat you have.

One interesting thing to note is that the further you move away from your body fat set point, the more severe the level of adaptation to a highly restricted caloric intake. Even though individual set points can vary greatly, one thing remains constant: the leaner you get, the worse the aforementioned problems become.

> This is why you can easily lose the first few pounds or kilos. But as you get leaner, and especially as you drop to lower depths of body fat, you will have extreme difficulty being able to burn off that stubborn fat.

This is why in the My Body Diet we use methods such as re-feeds, as it's shown in this study (17) by Friedl in the Journal of Applied Physiology that the use of a strategic re-feed, where calories and carbohydrates were raised, was able to prompt the recovery of metabolism with increased thyroid hormone, testosterone, and IGF-1.

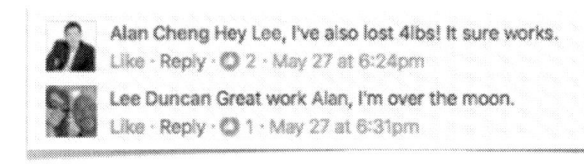

> Alan Cheng Hey Lee, I've also lost 4lbs! It sure works.
> Like · Reply · 2 · May 27 at 6:24pm
>
> Lee Duncan Great work Alan, I'm over the moon.
> Like · Reply · 1 · May 27 at 6:31pm

> Troy Zischke Love it Chris Dufey! You're the man with a wealth of knowledge! No other trainer/coach has been able to push me like this to get back on track to achieve my goals! Stay tuned people for the before and afters in the months to come!
> Like · Reply · 20 mins

Regular and properly used, refuel meals are an important step to not only giving your body what's needed on a physiological aspect so that you can be a fat burning machine, but I also believe there are important psychological aspects that help you. Because, if you know you will get to pig out on your favorite foods and chill out, you're much more likely to stay on track with the meal plan and enjoy the process.

In this study by Davoodi et al. (2014) (18), they compared the dieting method I use against the traditional dieting methods. The calorie cycling group had three days of no set calories and free living, eating what they wanted. This group lost more weight, even while they had 9 out of the 42 days completely free of any dieting and eating their favorite foods.

The other group that didn't have the re-feeds, also had a 50% higher amount of weight regain compared to the calorie cycling group. This science, along with the 1000's of men and women that have followed the meal plans and programs, shows that when you use a smarter diet, you're going to achieve much faster fat loss, enjoy the process, and be able to keep the weight off for long-term success.

This also shows that using the calorie and carb shifting method that we do in the My Body Diet, proper protein intake to suit you, along with the use of Metabolic Resistance Training, it is giving your brain and your body what's needed to avoid falling into the negative pitfalls that traditional dieting sets you up for. You are unique and an individual, and why you need your meal plan, workouts, lifestyle guidance, and entire plan crafted to suit you. And why a cookie-cutter, especially based on the wrong principles, is never going to give you the ultimate results you want.

That's why, in Part 2 of this book, I'm going to show you how to individualize the entire plan to suit you, and in such an easy to follow way that you're never going to be confused.

4

"CALORIES MATTER … I JUST DON'T COUNT THEM"

It is 6 am, and I'm sitting in a villa in Thailand on skype with Dr. Jade Teta. I'm interviewing Jade for the My Body Blends podcast, and I go straight for the throat!

I love every opportunity I get to talk with Jade, and this being his third time on the podcast, we wanted to delve straight into what the listeners really needed to understand and be doing to burn off stubborn fat.

Only minutes into our conversation, as we are peeling back our thoughts on how the connection of living a happy life, and being able to get in and stay in great shape can happen. Then he brilliantly sums it up with, "Calories matter. I just don't count them."

This wraps up perfectly how I feel with where the traditional weight loss advice has gone wrong. The 'count your calories' (so you can burn more energy than you eat) way to lose weight is flawed.

Don't get me wrong, I agree that the energy balance principle is important. Calories do matter. How much food you eat does play a big role in weight loss (or gain). However, counting calories to manage your energy intake is the wrong answer for so many people.

That's why shortly I'm going to be showing you the easy to use portion control guide so you can put down your calorie counting apps, stop the mental math, and ditch the food scales. But there's a simple reason this new method works so well, counting calories can derail you because it can not only be giving you the wrong information -- it's also giving you <u>too much</u> information.

This is why I love Nicola's transformation so much.

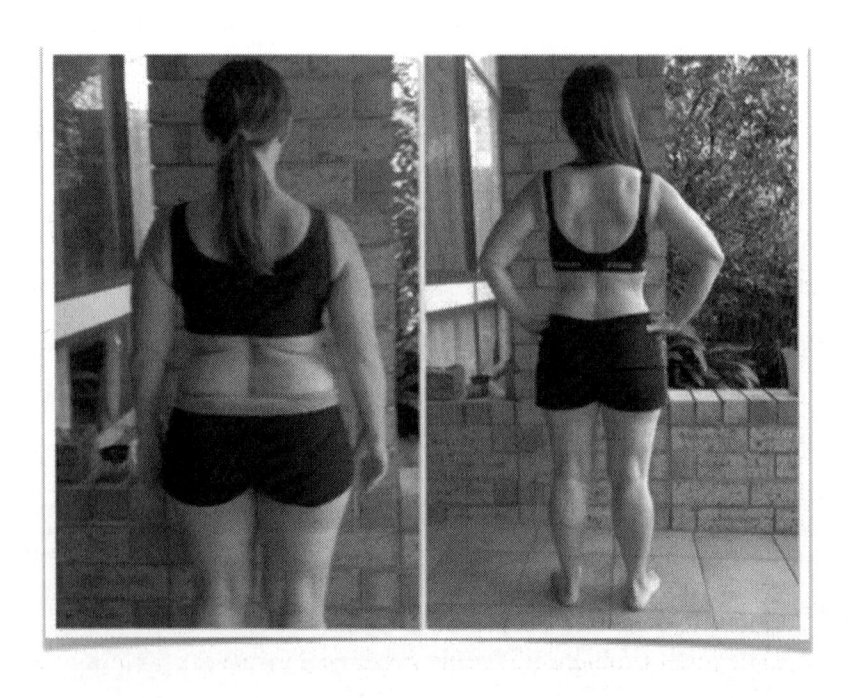

She was eating more and exercising less than what she was doing before she started our program. And as you can see, she was able to create a dramatic change in her body, especially with the common parts known as the "stubborn fat" areas. This is where we find those "hard to lose" areas of the body, such as hips, thighs, and butts for women, and lower back and belly fat for men. These can be the hardest bits to lose.

The main focus of writing this for you is to give you the real-world answer to taking back control of your body and health. And when you're trying to make changes in your life, especially when it involves our habits and behaviors around food and exercise, too much granular detail and conflicting information can make the change harder for you.

This is where we need to kill off the belief right now that you just need to follow the advice from most trainers, nutritionists, physicians along with the flood of blogs, magazines, books, and TV shows. And that advice is to stop being so lazy and go and exercise more, and stop being such a glutton and eat less food.

The fact is that 95% of people are failing at losing weight and keeping it off. Studies clearly show that when people try to lose weight by reducing the number of calories and amount of food they eat, they almost always lose weight in the short term. But then they follow up with weight gain over the next several months or years. These studies even show a large percentage of people are actually fatter two years after beginning a diet and exercise program than they were before it. (101)

The other problem this really highlights is that it's pointing the blame at you and your lack of willpower for not being able to follow the lower calorie diet. And I want to say to you right now is that if you've tried the whole traditional dieting approach and it hasn't worked for you: **It's not your fault.**

It's not your lack of willpower. And I will show you in a later chapter why trying to rely on just your willpower is a losing method. Your biology is stronger than your willpower.

The entire approach of restricted and forbidden foods is fundamentally flawed, and it sets people up for unhealthy relationships between themselves and food. This is why I'm going to turn you around from having a 'quantity' focused approach, that's constantly looking at "how much food am I allowed to eat?" to a 'quality' focused approach, which is a "what foods do I want to enjoy right now?"

Traci Mann, a UCLA associate professor and lead of the study, (102) put it well when she said, " We found that the majority of people regained all the weight, plus more. Sustained weight loss was found only in a small minority of participants, while complete weight regain, was found in the majority. Diets do not lead to sustained weight loss or health benefits for the majority of people."

Then co-author of the study, Janet Tomiyama, said, " Several studies indicate that dieting is actually a consistent predictor of future weight gain."

That pretty much sums up that if you want to struggle with weight loss and possibly even gain more weight, then you should follow the traditional dieting advice.

Apart from these reasons, I also find that there are three further reasons as to why counting calories is NOT going to get you the weight loss results you want, and how from here, you can be setting yourself up for further weight struggles by damaging your metabolism.

There are three reasons as I see that counting calories is flawed:

1. The calorie numbers vary up to 50%.
   The labeling of foods, and the wide range of databases that you use to calculate the energy density of foods can be off by up to 50%. It's also known that food companies can use up to five different methods to estimate calories, and that the FDA also allows errors of up to 20%.
2. Your foods change in calorie value depending on how you cook them.
   Chopping, blending, or cooking generally increases the availability of absorption, and this is not always reflected on the labeling of the foods.
   We absorb calories differently from person to person and from food to food.
3. Our gut health and microbiome (which I will show you how to fix soon) determine the absorption rate of calories along with macronutrients, and vitamins, and minerals. The problem is it's easy to see all the above as confusing, with the gross oversimplification that the idea that a gram of any protein yields 4 kcal, a gram of any fat yields 9 kcal, and a gram of any carbohydrate yields 4 kcal. This makes the calorie counting method to control energy balance

inaccurate.

The Low-Calorie Trap and Damaging Your Metabolism

The biggest problem is that your entire focus goes into the 'quantity' of food you are eating and the amount of exercise you are doing. As 'dieting,' for most of us, means eating less food and more gym when following the traditional weight loss advice.

The constant regurgitated advice of "you just need to be in a calorie deficit to lose weight" quickly leads to – a little is good, then a lot must be a better approach. This turns into a constant act of cutting out calories, cutting down on foods, and ramping up the amount of exercise you do. Especially, when on a week to week basis, you're NOT seeing your body change the way you want it to.

A great example of this is the common scenario I see with females that have competed in bikini or fitness model competitions. Their previous attempts to get 'stage and photo shoot ready lean' has had them following severe diets that have impacted their physiology and hormonal environment.

Through our skype call, I can tell they are frustrated with their lack of results from the weeks to months of sticking strictly to their diets, working hard, and yet, not getting lean. The biggest problem, though, is that they have dropped their food intake so low, and are exercising at such a high volume each day, that when you do the calorie calculation, they are in a much higher calorie deficit that they 'should' be.

(FYI – I will touch on the difference between men and women

and how they adapt and react differently to training, diet, and lifestyle changes).

All calories are created equal: Lie

The theory that the number of calories you consume versus calories you expend determines your weight loss is not a black and white answer. The science is far more complicated than that due to the fact that us humans are incredibly complex biological machines that science is still unraveling all the factors.

And this is why I'm going to walk you through in plain English, to clearly understand what REALLY matters when it comes to you burning off the unwanted weight, and even more importantly, what it is you can be doing day to day to get the body-changing results you want and still enjoy living your life.

Newton's first law of thermodynamics states that the energy of an isolated system is constant. This refers to a laboratory or a caloriebometer, which is an 'isolated system.' But this does not directly apply to our living, breathing, digesting human bodies. When you eat food, the 'isolated system' that creates the calorie equation goes out the window. The food interacts with your digestion, bacteria, and complex adaptive system that instantly transforms with each meal.

To give you a simple example of this, let's look at the difference between 500 calories of soft drink (or soda depending on where you live) and 500 calories of cauliflower.

When drinking the soft drink, you will quickly absorb the sugars, as there is a lack of fiber to go along with the sugar. Your blood sugar spikes, that then starts the flow-on effect of negative hormonal reactions. Increased insulin increases the storage of belly fat with extended exposure, and also increases inflammation, triglycerides, and blood pressure. (2)

But, this is where it can turn into a downward spiral. Your appetite increases, making you want to eat more, and because your blood sugar levels are now thrown out of whack (technical term), you crave more sugary foods. Then your appetite-controlling hormone, leptin, can become blocked, stopping the "I'm full" signal going back to the brain.

The high amount of fructose in the soft drink acts differently in your liver to glucose where it can further trigger more insulin resistance, making it harder for you to lose weight and priming you for later fat gain. There is also a further rise in inflammation, which can cause weight gain and diabetes and worsen your insulin resistance. Ghrelin, which is another 'hunger hormone,' goes up when you're hungry and down when you're satisfied from eating. One study (1) shows that fructose leads to higher ghrelin levels, which equals more hunger than glucose. Fructose also does not stimulate the satiety center in the brain (3) the same way glucose does, leading to a reduced feeling of being satisfied after eating. I, personally, have battled with the problem for years. It's the feeling that your stomach is full, yet your brain is telling you to keep eating more.

(Note: I will touch on later on the big difference between the small amount of fructose that comes from eating fruit in its whole form, compared to fructose that is used in processed foods. Fruit, in its whole form, is good food for you).

Now the other problem is the 500 calories from the soft drink is that we then end up with the common 'overfed and undernourished' setback. These are 'empty calories' because they are devoid of nutrition. There is no fiber, vitamins, or minerals to nourish your body.

Now let's take a look at what happens when you eat 500 calories of cauliflower. I've chosen cauliflower to be the other side of this example as both cauliflower and soft drinks are technically carbohydrates, and they both convert into sugars in the body. But the difference in these two foods has a profound difference to your body.

The obvious difference between 500 calories of soft drink to 500 calories of cauliflower is the volume of food, as I highly doubt you could fit in all that cauliflower in one or even two meals. But let's look at the physiological and hormone impact for now.

The amount of fiber means that much of the food isn't actually absorbed, and can positively lead to feeding the good bacteria in your gut, which you'll see soon in a later chapter why this is so important. The small amount of sugar in the cauliflower along with the high amount of fiber means that your blood sugars only rise a fraction. This means there is no crazy hormonal cascade. Your appetite hormones are kept under control, which means you feel full and satisfied and not cravings sugary foods.

The vitamins, minerals, and phytochemicals reduce inflammation, boost detoxification, and nourish your body with the nutrients it needs to thrive. And this can easily show the conclusion that —

- Not all calories are created equal.
- The response in your body is very different, and this is why I believe we need to look at the 'quality' of our foods before we start looking at the 'quantity' of our foods.

Why TEF Matters

The Thermic Effect of Food (TEF) shows us the difference in how different foods are metabolized in the body, and how different foods increase energy expenditure due to how our bodies digest, absorb, and metabolize the nutrients.

The Thermic Effect of the macronutrients are (4)

- Fat: 2-3%
- Carbs: 6-8%
- Protein: 25-30%

This means that 100 calories of protein wind up being 75 calories, while 100 calories of fat become 98 calories.

Studies also show that high-protein diets boost metabolism by up to 80 to 100 calories per day compared to lower protein diets (5, 6). This is why when I walk you through your meal plan and how to easily know what foods to eat, you will be starting with protein to add the 'metabolic advantage.'

We've talked about the difference in foods and how they impact with leptin and ghrelin, your hunger hormones. Then I've just shown the difference in how your body can metabolize foods, further throwing off the 'calorie calculate method for weight loss.'

But – one of the biggest problems is that so much of the (wrong) weight loss advice is focused on the wrong thing. You need a plan that you can easily understand, and even more easily use in day to day life. This is why traditional diets have failed us because one of the biggest killers of it is the hunger that comes with trying to follow those diets.

And the power of protein doesn't stop with just the increased metabolism. It's also been shown that protein is the most fulfilling macronutrient (7,8), and that by increasing your protein intake, you could be losing weight without counting calories or controlling portions (9,10).

This shows that we can give you a metabolic advantage by eating an adequate amount of protein to cause 'automatic' weight loss. All foods have a 'satiety index,' which is a rating based on several factors. The previous example comparing the soft drink to cauliflower shows that not only the hormonal impact is greatly different, but also, you can easily overeat one food over another.

Twice now, I've had Jonathan Bailor showcased on the show as his groundbreaking book, The Calorie Myth: How to Eat More, Exercise Less, Lose Weight and Live Better, proves by picking apart over 1200 studies that counting calories is unnecessary and misleading. It's time to change the way we think about weight loss. Jonathan exposes the fundamental myths upon which the diet industry has been built: the eat less + exercise more = weight loss equation.

Bailor has conceptualized his SANE calorie qualities – Satiety, Aggression (whether calories will be stored as body fat), Nutrition, and Efficiency (how those calories are stored). These must all be in balance to achieve optimum results.

In 2004, a study (11) conducted by Yancy et al. for the Annals of Internal Medicine concluded as follows:

Compared with a low-fat diet, **a low-carbohydrate diet program had better participant retention and greater weight loss.**

So, <u>what</u> you eat (rather than simply how much you eat) can not only affect your weight, it can also affect the likelihood of you sticking to a particular eating regime.

Now, don't get me wrong. I'm not saying that calories don't matter. It's just there is a much smarter and easier way than forcing yourself to restrict the amount of food and, therefore, the number of calories you eat, to get you to lose unwanted weight.

This is why we now need to look into the power of your hormones and how your hormones are affecting how and where you are losing or gaining weight from.

5
WHY HORMONES MATTER

You losing fat and building muscle shows up on the outside. But how well or how quickly you're able to have this happen is determined by what happens on the inside.

This is why I'm going to simply have you understand how your hormones can flick the 'switch' for your body storing fat, or burning fat, with other hormones playing vital roles that dictate your hunger, cravings, metabolism, energy, mental clarity, and mood.

When Kansas state professor, Mark Haub, went from 33% body fat to 25% body fat by only Twinkies, this backed up that just eating fewer calories is all that mattered.

The counting calories model for weight loss is a simple addition and subtraction model, and even though the model is flawed, it's easy for your brain to grasp the concept. The problem with understanding hormones is that they're not as easy to 'count.'

Yes! We can certainly, and I do recommend, get blood, urine, and saliva testing done that will report on your hormonal levels. But it's as simple as if your testosterone is at 600, then you are burning a certain amount of fat each day. We have good ranges for which your hormonal lab testing should be in for optimal health and function. Though I want to walk you through how you can achieve lasting fat loss through balanced hormonal environment.

Your body can regulate how much food you take in by controlling your hunger. By also controlling your metabolism, it can regulate how many calories you are expending. But if we look at people who are overweight and obese, we can clearly see that something is out of whack (there's that technical terminology again).

Because these people are over consuming calories, you would expect them to have faster metabolisms and to not have any issues with hunger from the amount of food that is being consumed. But here is the problem; people who are overweight or obese nearly always have the opposite; high hunger and a slow metabolism.

This can be related to "leptin resistance." And I'm going to walk you through in just a minute three of the major hormonal imbalances that could be causing you to gain weight and struggle to lose weight.

Before we do that, let's get a firm grasp on the important metabolism hormones and how they are controlling your fat loss, hunger, mood, and more…

Insulin: This is one of the most misunderstood hormones, it's been the victim of a bashing over the past years. Insulin is a powerful 'storage' hormone where it is mainly produced when you eat carbohydrates, and mildly when eating protein. High insulin levels can often mean fat storage from excessive eating. Insulin also blunts the body's ability to burn fat for fuel.

So, the low-carb movement came from focusing mainly on cutting back carbs so that you have a lowered insulin response. There is a lot of merit behind this, though like many things in the health and nutrition world, it was taken too far. Very low-carb diets became the diet to follow, and there are issues when following these types of plans. Especially, when they are too drastic or followed for too long.

I will be walking you through the 'priming phase' that I use as a reset button for members and clients so that you can get the best starting plan, and we do use a 'smart carb' approach to accelerate your fat burning.

The goal is to make your body more insulin sensitive. When insulin sensitivity is high, you need less insulin to achieve the same effect. High insulin sensitivity is one of the best ways to ensure you can burn body fat, and therefore, use carbs to fuel your recovery and muscle growth.

Most diets just try to cut out carbs to then limit and control insulin, though there is a backlash effect that can happen when you cut carbs by too much and for too long. This can reverse insulin sensitivity to more insulin resistance, lowering metabolic hormones, such as thyroid, and also making you a grouch of a person when you're constantly struggling with increased hunger and cravings.

This is why I'm going to show you how to exercise properly, so that you increase your insulin sensitivity, and how you can easily go each day and week eating foods that control your insulin levels, prevent a constant rollercoaster of highs and lows, and also use your favorite carb foods to cause high insulin spikes at the right times so that you can increase fat burning and hormonal balance.

The other great use of insulin is that it helps to control hunger and build muscle. Even you ladies that are reading this, you want to be able to harness the positive effects of insulin. And why as both male and female client's I want you to use a plan that takes everything into account, rather than missing out by being misinformed as so many people do.

Leptin: Have you or have you seen a friend ever drop lots of weight initially, and then struggle with the final 5 to 10 pounds?

A big part of this issue can be linked back to leptin, as this hormone is produced in your fat cells. This is why it can be easier to drop weight when you have more excess body fat to lose.

Your leptin levels tell your brain how your 'fuel' and fat levels are. Excessive dieting or radical plans can disrupt your leptin levels and cause metabolic compensation. Leptin can also be linked to your caloric intake. So when you eat fewer calories, your leptin levels drop, and this can then lower other fat burning hormones.

The less leptin you produce, the hungrier you become. This then creates a catch-22, as you need to eat less to burn fat. But then by eating less, you produce less leptin. Making it harder and harder for you to keep losing weight.

One common issue is 'leptin resistance,' where your brain loses the ability to pick up on the leptin's signal and has you overeating. This is what we see in overweight and obese individuals, where the hunger 'switch' seems to be broken and always turned on.

Thyroid: Can be seen as your metabolism's thermostat, as it strongly impacts your energy levels.

Low-calorie and/or low-carbohydrate diets are what can impact your leptin and thyroid levels and then, in turn, bring about the 'metabolic slowdown' that makes your weight loss near impossible.

Thyroid is also linked with stress, and this is why we can take back control through the changes in lifestyle; decreasing the stress of low-calorie dieting and smarter training.

Human Growth Hormone: You've probably heard of Human Growth Hormone (HGH) as the elixir of youth and anti-aging hormone. This hormone has powerful effects on your body's ability to burn body fat and mildly on building muscle.

One reason why, in the plan, I have you focusing on good quality sleep, using small bouts of fasting, and smarter Metabolic Resistance Training, and why the meal plan and phases are set up so that you can produce greater Growth Hormone.

Cortisol: This is another hormone that has got a bad rap. It's been bashed as our modern-day lives mean it's easy to fall into the trap of having excessively high and prolonged exposure to cortisol. This powerful hormone can help, or impede, your fat burning, and like many things; "the poison's in the dose."

This is why we want to bring about balance, it's not about trying to shut all cortisol off, we want to use the effects it can have as a positive and accelerate your fat burning, but not have too much where it can slow down weight loss or even help in fat storage.

This is why we want to create the 'environment' so your body can thrive. When cortisol is produced with testosterone and HGH, for example when training properly, it can certainly aid and accelerate the fat burning process. If it's produced with low testosterone and HGH, such as when you're stressed day to day, not eating or moving properly, this can aid the fat storage process.

Cortisol is one the body's stress hormones. And the common misconception about cortisol is that it's not just 'lifestyle stress,' such as running late for work that can cause you to have excessive cortisol, nutritional stress, such as underrating or undernourishment, food allergies or sensitivities, emotional stress, over-training, undersleeping, and recovery all come onto the scene when causing your body to produce cortisol.

Testosterone: For you guys reading right now, this is scary.

Over the past 20 years, the average male's testosterone has dropped from 20-30%. And this can directly cause problems for you not being able to burn the fat, build the muscle, have the confidence to act the way you want.

Testosterone helps improve the ability for you to build muscle, have higher insulin sensitivity, and maintain metabolic health. Most diets don't take testosterone into account when they tell you to eat low amounts of fat - especially, the saturated and monounsaturated fats that help boost testosterone, and exercise is the wrong way that can lower your levels and not boost it.

For you ladies reading, testosterone is still important for you. Higher amounts of testosterone in relation to the balance of estrogen and progesterone thicken the waist and lead to a more apple-shaped body. This is why when it comes to testosterone and all hormones, it's not just a matter of amount, but of having the right balance.

This is why we've designed everything from the workouts to meal plans, to improving your sleep, lifestyle, and stress and are all created with your hormonal balance in mind.

Estrogen: Both men and women need estrogen, it's just that women need higher levels. For both sexes, estrogen is tied to your ability to burn fat, build muscle, and control hunger.

An example of this is the relationship between estrogen and the brain chemicals GABA (gamma-aminobutyric acid), serotonin, and dopamine. When a woman is going through her menstrual cycle, her hunger, cravings, mood, and energy can change due to the changes in estrogen and its relationship to the brain chemicals.

Estrogen can be a fat storing and burning hormone. It can help with insulin sensitivity and in blocking the negative effects of cortisol. It is also linked to stubborn fat storage for women on the hips, thighs, and butt. An imbalance for men can cause 'man-boobs' (gynecomastia) and contribute to increasing the risk of prostate cancer and heart disease. It can also cause lower testosterone levels, which develop further issues, such as I mentioned above.

We will also cover other hormones such as ghrelin, adrenaline, and neuropeptide-Y throughout the book as I take you through how to shape the body of your dreams.

What you are going to learn and use from this book are the guiding principles and plans for you to use simply, so that you have the proper hormonal balance, can naturally control your food intake, and allow you to turn into a fat burning machine that's healthy.

6

BIG 3 HORMONAL IMBALANCES

There are 'biochemical forces' that make us eat more and exercise less.

The fitness and weight loss industry has been focused on the presumption of weight loss is due to people eating too much, and not moving enough. Basically, that the behavior and lack of willpower causing the behavior is the problem.

This is why when we look at the 3 big hormone imbalances that are so common, it clearly shows us that these 'forces,' which are causing you to struggle to lose weight, are not to do with your lack of willpower.

The Blood Sugar Rollercoaster

The pendulum still swings to and fro when it comes to eating sugar and if it really is bad for you or not. However, let's just focus on what matters here and how insulin, the bodies 'storage' hormone, can be one of the biggest problems in your weight struggles if you don't follow a few key principles.

When eating too much sugar or carbohydrates, regular high spikes of insulin that are produced to try and ferry them out of the blood and into tissue. With constant exposure, your cells can be desensitized to insulin. This is what we call 'insulin resistance,' and it is why so many millions of people (and possibly yourself) struggle to lose weight. If that wasn't bad enough, too much sugar in the blood is also linked to an increase in triglycerides (fats) in the blood, which raise your risk of heart disease, it can ruin your arteries and nerves, and be linked to type 2 diabetes.

Insulin resistance also actives lipogenic (fat-forming) genes in your liver, which can result in even more sugar and free fatty acids being converted into fat. It can also cause an enzyme process in the liver to be prone to converting excess sugar into fat.

Then we have the other side of the 'blood sugar rollercoaster,' and that is when it reduces. This is when you have low blood sugar levels, known as hypoglycemia. This can lead to an increase of inflammation and also the production of cortisol. It's cortisol's job to increase blood sugar levels. When you have blood sugar lows, the famous 'hangry' state can rear its ugly head, even out of the nicest people. This is when you're hungry and angry at the same time because your low blood sugar levels are needing you to eat something to stabilize your levels quickly.

This is when you can easily start reaching for the foods that you know aren't the best choices.

The typical 'western diet' day can show you how this happens.

For breakfast, you have toast, orange juice, or even some fruit and granola. This is a high carb, low protein, and low-fat breakfast, which will quickly produce a high insulin response, that soon after, cause your blood sugars to drop. So, at about 10am, you're starving again, and with your now low blood sugar levels, you're reaching for a coffee and a muffin for a quick pick me up of energy.

(Now, I love coffee, and I see many benefits of it. But reaching for coffee just for the stimulant effect, and especially with a high-carb meal, can be a recipe for disaster if it becomes a habit).

You have lunch of maybe a sandwich, and then by 3pm, you hit the famous mid-afternoon slump of energy. You're dead tired and are on the hunt for some sugary, energy giving foods to get you through the rest of the afternoon. By the time dinner rolls around, your entire day has been a rollercoaster of ups and downs for your blood sugars. This doesn't even take into account how our modern, and stressful lives can further affect your blood sugars by the overproduction of stress from lifestyle factors.

Now to make matters worse, increased insulin levels can upregulate an enzyme called aromatase, which in men, will convert their testosterone to estrogen. The opposite reaction occurs in women and can cause low estrogen and too high a level of testosterone.

Increased insulin levels can also be tied into elevating your leptin levels, which can further lead to 'leptin resistance,' where just like insulin resistance, the leptin signal to the brain becomes 'numb,' and your brain doesn't pick up on the signals.

Then we also have the problem of increased inflammation from an increase of a chemical called interleukin-6 (IL-6), which can further raise cortisol and have other damaging effects on the body. Finally, insulin can impair your ability to detox toxins and excess hormones out of the body by weakening your liver's ability to do its job properly. This can lead to having to a high level of estrogen in the body, further increasing fat storage and upregulating alpha-adrenergic receptors and causing stubborn fat.

(note: I'm going to walk you through the 'stubborn fat fix' later in this book, and you will see how you DO NOT want upregulation of alpha-androgenic receptors).

Now the above paints a real crap-storm of a picture, but this is not all doom-and-gloom. You just need to understand that the body does not work in a vacuum when it comes to hormones that are impacting each other. This is why a holistic view is needed, and why, when you follow the My Body Diet, you're going to create the balance needed, so that you look, feel, and function the way you want each day.

We do this by first resetting your body with the Priming Phase, and then each step after focuses on creating hormonal balance that further positively affects each other.

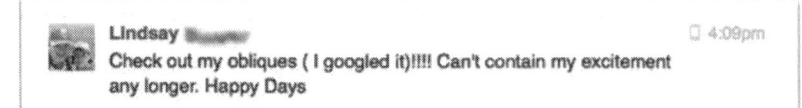

> **Lindsay** 4:09pm
> Check out my obliques (I googled it)!!!! Can't contain my excitement any longer. Happy Days

The Stress Fat Factor

We've already talked about cortisol and how it can have a negative effect when in overproduction and kept high for too long. Cortisol is, however, not all bad, we do need it, and it does have some very positive effects on the body. One of which, when produced at the right time and with low insulin levels, can help your body go through the fat burning process.

However, our bodies and brains are not wired for the modern-day lives that we live. Our bodies are made to perceive a threat and then deal with it. Fantastically put in the great book; Why zebras don't get ulcers, Robert Sapolsky shows how when we don't deal with stress properly, it can have a host of terrible effects on our body. When a zebra gets stressed because she just saw a lion creeping up on her, her fight or flight mechanisms kick in. This involves a production of cortisol along with other stress sympathetic nervous system reactions. This helps the zebra run away.

Then, soon after as the zebra knows that she's safe, the stress hormones come back down to a normal level. We are not very dissimilar, though we are getting a constant flood of stress responses that can come from; being caught up in traffic and being late for work, financial stress, relationship stress, or even stress through nutrition, lack of sleep or toxicity.

This constant flood of problems that are causing a stress response means that you aren't able to properly deal with it, and it has the knock-on effect of causing harm in the body.

The major reasons too much cortisol impairs your ability to lose fat are:

- Having constant high blood sugar levels through the constant stimulation that high cortisol creates, which we know from above leads to fat storage.
- Creates an imbalance with leptin and can further exacerbate the problem that causes leptin resistance, so your brain doesn't get the "I'm full" signal, and you can easily over eat.
- Lower your thyroid hormone, especially the active form, which is T3, by decreasing your body's ability to convert it. This slows your metabolism further.
- Lowers your ability to use insulin, which again, from what we covered above, we know can lead to fat storage and make it harder for your body to burn fat for fuel.
- Can affect your gut health and microbiome, which can lead to problems of not being able to digest and absorb the nutrients you eat, and also, as you will soon see in a coming chapter on gut health, this can be directly related to fat storage.

This is why, when following the My Body Diet, it's NOT just a meal plan or traditional diet. It gives you the simple to follow meals and guidelines, the workouts, the nutrients, and the lifestyle factors that all need to be working together to bring about the balance of your hormones and create the environment for you to be a fat burning machine that can conquer each day.

According to a 30-year study conducted by Harvard, it's NOT increased food potions that make us fat.

The Harvard researcher believes that the behavior, increased food intake, and decreased exercise is **secondary** to changes in the function of hormones. (12)

It turns out that there are well defined biological mechanisms that can explain how the **foods** we eat disrupt the function of our **hormones**, which makes us eat more and gain weight (13). This shows us that the problem is that we're not getting fat because we're eating more, we're eating more because we're getting fat.

For example, with leptin resistance (put simply), the brain doesn't "see" the leptin. It doesn't see that we have enough fat stored, and therefore, thinks that we're starving. This is known as leptin resistance and is believed to be a leading driver of obesity (14).

If leptin doesn't work properly, your brain doesn't get the message, and you continue eating beyond your body's energy needs. We're eating more because the brain doesn't see the leptin and thinks we're starving. Trying to exert willpower against the leptin-driven starvation signal is next to impossible.

In broad strokes, the more fat you have, the more leptin you make and the less food you'll eat. And then vice versa, the less fat you have, the less leptin you produce and the more you want to eat.

This is commonly seen with bikini and fitness models. A usual preparation will have these athletes progress to a low-calorie diet and high exercise level. The metabolic adaptations that occur with the body 'fighting back' against the diet and exercise plan mean there is a "fat overshoot."

During the diet, the body will make the metabolic adaptations that make it harder to stick to a deprivations style diet. Then when the diet is over, a degree of leptin resistance is caused, along with a host of other issues that can cause the person to continually eat and not feel full. With the slowed metabolism and actual ability to create more fat cells in this state, the person can gain fat rapidly, and even gain more fat than what they had before they started the diet and exercise plan.

This issue can also be seen in overweight and obese individuals, as regardless of how much they eat, their brain can still think they are starving because as far as its concerned, it still thinks it's starving from there not being a high enough leptin signal.

When leptin and the body are working as they should, you will eat when you're hungry and not eat when you're full.

Then we have the common culprit, insulin, and how it relates to leptin. According to Dr. Lustig, one of the ways that insulin contributes to obesity, is by blocking the leptin signal in the brain (15).

With high insulin levels, you have a lowered leptin signal. So your brain thinks you're starving and low on energy, in turn, you get signals sent back to make you eat more. And with the already high insulin levels, it sends signals to the fat cells telling them to store fat and to hold on to the fat that they already carry (16).

This is why we want to reduce inflammation in the body and

reduce the foods that can be causing leptin issues in the first place. Also, by using a food cycling method that is one of the underlying principles the My Body Diet works by, we are able to have the right amount of food intake that will allow your body to burn body fat at an accelerated rate. But also balance the important metabolic hormones, such as leptin. By eating your favorite foods, such as ice cream, burgers, etc. so that you increase leptin levels and keep the fat burning fire ignited.

As the power of reducing inflammation was brilliantly highlighted to me by Dr. Barry Sears, author of many popular books, one being the Zone Diet, which was one of the first books I read when I was sick and tired of being fat and had to do something about it.

So you can imagine that being able to interview him multiple times was a total dream come true. But it was also the teaching he was able to pass on, in which how we are able to lower inflammation through our foods, lifestyle, and supplementation that has been a huge influencer on me designing the My Body Diet and our programs.

This is why, when you follow the My Body Diet, it's going to have you:

1. Actually burn fat and lose the unwanted weight.
2. Cause fat loss, by not forcibly depriving yourself of food when you're hungry. Instead, it causes fat loss by effortlessly driving the body to be in a state of burning more fat and limiting fat storage.

3. Fits in with your life to become a habit, so you can happily get on with your life and enjoy the body and health changing results.
4. Enhances cellular and hormonal health so you can easily keep the weight off.

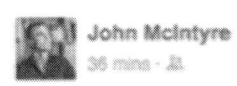

> **John McIntyre**
> 36 mins ·
>
> Shout out to my man Chris Dufey, the most ripped Aussie I've met.
>
> He just set me up with a detailed program to turn myself into the Hulk, and he's been super helpful with all the questions I've been asking.
>
> If you're looking to get in shape, whether by losing fat, building muscle, or both at the same time, talk to Chris. He'll also give you pointers on how to heal your adrenals with 1 "weird" morning drink trick (h/t Kurt), what supplements to take at what time of the day, and how to breathe for maximum results in and out of the gym.
>
> Message him now, tell him what you need and he'll sort you out.

Is Your Brain Making You Fat?

Your brain is in control of what is going on with your body. We've already walked through with how your hormones are the signals getting sent throughout your body, which are then telling your body whether to burn or store fat, be hungry or feel satisfied, want to go and exercise or feel tired and lay on the couch, and a host of other things that have a direct relationship with you being able to, or not being able to get in the body shape you want.

So, it's the health of your brain and its ability to talk to the rest of your body that is sitting in the driver's seat when it comes to your ability to lose weight. Where most diets and weight loss plan fail, is to take into account the importance of brain health and what it is that you can be doing to give yourself an unfair advantage to get into great shape.

What really shocked me was when I was interviewing Dr. Vera Tarman for the My Body Blends podcast as we were discussing eating addictions and disorders. It was only minutes into recording the interview, and I had to jump in and interrupt Dr. Vera.

"From what you're saying Vera, most of the health and fitness industry has an eating disorder?"

The answer was a resounding yes. And this is a huge issue that most people are completely ignoring and have no idea is going on.

If you've ever tried to cut back on the junk foods that you know you should be eating less of, you would have noticed the cravings that can kick in. Even though, logically, you know that the foods aren't that great for you, and they aren't going to help you get the body you want, some other part of the brain disagrees, and you find yourself finishing off the whole cookie jar (yes, I've certainly done this plenty of times).

The biggest issue I find with this falling to temptations and cravings is that you don't even really enjoy eating the foods because you're feeling guilty. And this guilty feeling continues on, and even with your best intentions, you find you can be doing it repeatedly.

Firstly, I want to tell you it's not your fault or your lack of willpower. We have unlimited access to foods now that are engineered to be hyperpalatable and are able to stimulate the reward center of your brain.

The brain knows that when you eat, you're doing something good. It releases 'feel good chemicals,' one of which is the neurotransmitter, dopamine. And we can be hardwired to go and search for behaviors that have us release dopamine (so we feel good).

The issue is that these engineered foods that are hyperpalatable, have a much stronger stimulation of your reward center and produce more dopamine. Eating a steak and sweet potato sure is scrumptious and will have a dopamine effect. But scooping your favorite choc chip cookies into Ben and Jerrys is going to have a much larger dopamine effect.

Then the problem continues as the brain can start to become numb to the dopamine effect. So, therefore, you need to have more of the foods to get the same 'feel good' effect.

This is where we need to talk about cravings. As this is an emotional state and is not the same as the feeling of hunger and the body needing energy. When you've tried to diet before, and you've wanted to cut out certain foods. You will often have cravings start from a certain cue. A habit or behavior that you're in is what gives you the cue to eat a certain food.

This is where craving is about satisfying your need for dopamine. And this can become totally overwhelming and take up your complete attention.

A common scenario is that you go through a normal day. It's busy, and you've been dealing with the daily responsibilities of your modern life. Throughout the day, you've been making smart food choices. You said no to the muffin at the mid-morning work meeting and opted for a green tea and apple. You pushed the bread basket away and enjoyed your salad for lunch.

By the time dinner rolls around, you've flexed your willpower muscle throughout the entire day. You're tired, and you're want to unwind at the end of the day. And this is where the craving for some chocolate (or insert your favorite food) comes crashing down on you. You try to fight it and ignore it. But eventually you cave, and before you know it, you've finished the whole block and think "I've ruined the whole day."

I don't believe this is emotionally or psychologically healthy, and I want to kill off people feeling bad about themselves when it comes to food.

"I'll just start again on Monday."

The famous words of so many people for when they do cave into cravings and temptations and have to wait until Monday for the same reset button to start all over again. This is where falling to cravings can turn into all-out binges and what could have been harmless, now turns into a fall-gaining tidal wave.

One example that is burned into my brain was a consultation I had with a 200kg man. A super successful businessman that, over the years, had got himself into a state where he had to choose carefully which restaurants he dines at, so they have big enough chairs for him to actually fit into. We got to the part of the consultation where I needed to understand from a psychological standpoint what got him to his current weight.

He talked me through that when times became stressful, either with relationships or with his business, then he would stop on the way home, or have bags of peanut M&Ms and pints of his favorite Hargendaas ice cream delivered. He would then hit the couch, pour the M&Ms into the ice cream and finish the whole thing. This could easily then turn into days-in-a-row of multiple binge-eating efforts.

The point is, you don't need to be struggling with cravings or even feeling bad, when we can nourish you with the right foods, bring about hormonal balance, create the brain health needed, and turn you into a fat burning machine.

The truth is, there's a smarter way than relying on willpower.

Think of willpower as a battery. At the start of the day, you've a full battery. But each and every decision you take takes a chunk of willpower energy away. Constantly making 'good' decisions throughout the day is going to dwindle your battery.

This is why at the end of the day, it's so easy to cave into your cravings. And especially when you've already set up the behavior and habit of eating dessert and having a wine with dinner.

Willpower may get you through a moment, but it's not the best strategy for permanently ending habits or addictions, or for making any lasting change for that matter. The effects of willpower are immediate, but not necessarily sustainable.

When I white knuckle, my way through a "no, thank you" to ice cream, that's helpful at that moment only. It does nothing to help me the next night. If I want to say no the next night, I need to summon up the energy and resolve at that moment--and it does take energy and resolve. Hopefully, the energy and resolve are available to me when I need them. Often, they aren't, which makes willpower not always possible.

When I work with people who want to stop binge eating, willpower doesn't cut it. While it may work on my little ice cream cravings, it is no match for the hijacking urges that accompany a serious habit. In the midst of an intense drive to binge eat (or smoke, drink, watch porn, or any of the habits I help people break), willpower doesn't stand a chance as a long-term strategy.

Hijacked by an urge, or in the middle of a deeply ingrained behavior is when you are least likely to have the resources you need to fight.

Willpower can get you over a hump or through a moment. It can help you decrease your nightly ice cream "habit" and get you out of bed some mornings. But it's not going to be of much help for the bigger things. It's simply too much work, requiring too much effort, for too little long-term impact.

And this is why there needs to be a set of steps that will have you setting up the habits and behaviors, so your success is set on autopilot. Setting up habits is all about having small steps setup so that it is easy for you to follow. This is why we focus on only ever creating and replacing one habit at a time.

This is also why we create 'sticky habits,' so that it makes use of your current routines instead of trying to fight old habits to replace new ones. Also, by limiting options and making things much simpler for yourself, you don't eat away at your willpower 'battery.'

After reading Charles Duhigg's best-selling book, The Power of Habit. He clearly outlines how we can use the three R's of habit change.

1. Reminder (the trigger that initiates the behavior)
2. Routine (the behavior itself; the action you take)
3. Reward (the benefit you gain from doing the behavior)

For lasting change, the steps you take must ultimately <u>change your environment</u> and schedule. Stop buying snacks if you want to stop snacking (no willpower needed), pack a similar lunch every day of the week, and embrace the power of routine to get the necessary done each day.

I know…

It's not sexy. But, it works really well! And it's by having to go through the steps myself and then watching 1000's of others that have used the same process, that I have refined it to make it the best possible. You can be setting yourself up for success on autopilot

Now that we covered how you are going to win the battle against cravings and set yourself up for automatic success and not rely on willpower, you need to understand how your gut health and brain are connected.

How serotonin and other neurotransmitters are found in the gut

How to Fix Your Gut Bacteria and Lose Weight

We've only recently started to get a grasp and understand the huge importance and role that your gut bacteria plays in health and disease. As the mind-bending fact is that there are ten times more bacteria than the sum total of all the cells in the body.

We know that the composition and makeup of your gut microbiome play a role in how your body stores the food you eat, how easy it is for you to lose weight, and how well your metabolism functions.

Researchers have also shown that gut micro biome "play an unexpectedly important role in exacerbated post-dieting weight gain, and that this common phenomenon may, in the future, be prevented or treated by altering the composition or function of the microbiome." (19)

What first really grabbed my attention with this is that the study showing that mice without a protein known as toll-like receptor 5 (TLR5) in their gut gain excessive weight and develop diabetes. But what was really shocking is that when researchers transferred the gut flora from the overweight mice into skinny mice, they immediately started eating more, becoming overweight, and developing metabolic abnormalities. (20)

People who struggle to maintain a healthy weight after dieting may do so because their gut bacteria retains a "memory" of their past weight, according to scientists.

The study, in mice, suggests that yo-yo dieting is not simply a reflection of people returning to unhealthy eating habits, but could be driven by long-term changes in gut bacteria brought about by obesity. (19)

Dr. Steve Gundry which has been one of the worlds preeminent experts in heart surgeon is also the author of The Plant Paradox. He further opened my eyes to the importance of our mitochondria and microbiome.

With regard to mitochondria, "mitochondrial flexibility is one of the unique things that make us human," Gundry says.

"The reason we're designed to [store fat is to] be able to access fat for fuel," Gundry says. *"The reason why [humans] have been able to take over all parts of the world ... [is] because we can cycle back and forth, having our mitochondria use fat for fuel or glucose for fuel. We're designed to shift very quickly ... even within 24 hours.*

[Most people] no longer have that metabolic flexibility [because] we've been constantly bombarding our mitochondria with an overload of glucose as a fuel, and that really underlies, I think, most disease processes."

This is also why we use intermittent fasting as one of the strategies to fast track your health and weight loss. So you can easily have an eating window that suits your body and lifestyle to help improve your "metabolic flexibility".

Eran Elinav, an immunologist at the Weizmann Institute in Israel and lead author, said "It may explain some – more than some – of our failure to control weight by dieting."

How this relates directly to you and me is that this is another factor that is not about willpower, or anyone struggling with weight loss being lazy or a glutton. It's that you can have forces working against you that can be making it much harder for you to lose weight, and even prone to gaining fat.

There are now studies, such as ""Fecal Microbiota Transplant for Obesity and Metabolism" (21) that are testing to see if transplanting the intestinal bacteria from a healthy, lean person into the gut of a person suffering from obesity can change the gut bacteria population of that obese person. As those "lean microbes" start to populate the obese person's gut, it could reduce that person's propensity to obesity.

Or, in plain English, we're talking about capsules that contain a tiny amount of human poo from a thin person could make you thin. The lead researcher, Elaine W. Yu, an assistant professor at Harvard Medical School and a clinical researcher at Massachusetts General Hospital, said, "A small study in humans has already been done that demonstrates that altering gut bacteria affects human metabolism."

It could be the reason for how changes in the gut flora can cause diabetes is that a different species of bacteria seems to have different effects on appetite and metabolism. Other studies have shown that changes in the gut flora can increase the rate at which we absorb fatty acids and carbohydrates, and also increase the storage of calories as fat. This means that someone with bad gut flora could eat the same amount of food as someone with a healthy gut, but extract more calories from it and gain more weight. (22)

Being a dad, I enjoy geeking out and being able to give my children the absolute best ability to achieve what they want in life. And one way this relates directly is that we also know that infants that are not breastfed are more likely to develop unhealthy gut bacteria. And these gut bacteria changes early on in life may predict being overweight or even obese in the future (23).

Dominguez-Bello, for example, is conducting a clinical trial in Puerto Rico in which babies born by cesarean section are immediately swabbed with a gauze cloth laced with the mother's vaginal fluids and resident microbes. She will track the weight and overall health of the infants in her study, comparing them with C-section babies who did not receive the gauze treatment.

What all of these fun facts show, is that having healthy gut bacteria is crucial to maintaining normal weight and metabolism. And this can become a real issue as the modern lifestyle has a few problems that contribute to unhealthy gut flora.

Things like; antibiotic use, eating too much refined carbohydrates and sugars, not eating enough fermentable fibers, dietary toxins, and even chronic stress.

Optimal gut balance begins with your diet, which directly affects that balance. You want to eat a diet with lots of fiber, healthy protein, and healthy fats.

Good fats, including Omega 3 fats and monounsaturated fats – such as extra-virgin olive oil, avocados or almonds – improve healthy gut flora, while inflammatory fats, such as Omega 6 and vegetable oils promote the growth of bad bugs that cause weight gain and disease.

Yes, inflammatory fats will definitely damage your gut bacteria. But the right fats, including Omega 3s and extra-virgin olive oil combined with a whole, real-food diet can actually repair your gut and even increase good bacteria.

This is exactly why I designed the My Body Diet and all the steps I have for you to follow easily; help remove toxins from the diet, add in fermentable fibers, reduce inflammation, manage stress, and set you up for a healthy gut.

The recommendations I make to do with your gut health are not miracle cures. They are the actions that lead to normalized gut function and flora through improved diet, increased fiber intake, daily probiotic supplementation, the use of nutrients that repair the gut lining.

From your very first breath, you are exposed to probiotics.

A newborn on its way through the birth canal during a natural delivery is dosed with the bacteria from the mother. And this is what starts the bacterial colonization in the infant's gastrointestinal (GI) tract.

Compelling new research now shows many cesarean section infants have less-than-optimal health after birth. This is most likely because they are not exposed to the mother's bacteria in the birth canal, which would then serve to populate its own GI tract.

Are you getting enough probiotic-rich foods in your diet? Chances are, you're probably not. Probiotics are good bacteria that primarily line your gut and are responsible for nutrient absorption and supporting your immune system.

If you don't have enough probiotics, the side effects can include: digestive disorders, skin issues, candida, autoimmune disease, and frequent colds and flu.

Historically, we had plenty of probiotics in our diet from eating fresh foods from good soil, and by fermenting our foods to keep them from spoiling.

However, today, because of refrigeration and dangerous

agricultural practices like soaking our foods with chlorine, our food contains little to no probiotics, and most foods today actually contain antibiotics that kill off the good bacteria in our bodies.

By adding more probiotic foods into your diet, you could see all of the following health benefits:

- Stronger immune system
- Improved digestion
- Increased energy from production of vitamin B12
- Better breath because probiotics destroy candida
- Healthier skin, since probiotics improve eczema and psoriasis
- Reduced cold and flu
- Healing from leaky gut and inflammatory bowel disease
- Weight loss

Sound good? If you want all of these benefits, then it's time to start consuming these probiotic foods for better health. In fact, you should eat a variety of types of probiotics, as each one offers a different type of beneficial bacteria to help the body in a variety of ways.

For a long time, scientists considered gut bacteria essentially as digestive aids, but we now know that the variety and quantity of bacteria affect our overall health and wellbeing in a number of ways.

Top 4 Probiotic Foods

1. Cultured vegetables - Sauerkraut and kimchi

Made from fermented cabbage and other vegetables, sauerkraut is not diverse in probiotics but is high in organic acids, which give food its sour taste and support the growth of good bacteria. Sauerkraut is extremely popular in Germany today. Kimchi is a cousin to sauerkraut and is the Korean take on cultured veggies. Both of the fermented formulas are also high in enzymes, which can aid digestion. They contain some probiotics, but also, they contain certain types of acids like gluconic acid and acetic acid, healthy acids that create a certain type of pH in your body that supports the growth of probiotics in your system.

2. Coconut Kefir

    Made by fermenting the juice of young coconuts with kefir grains, this dairy-free option for kefir has some of the same probiotics as traditional dairy kefir but is typically not as high in probiotics. Still, it has several strains that are beneficial for your health.

3. Kombucha

    Is an effervescent fermentation of black tea that is started by using a SCOBY, also known as a symbiotic colony of bacteria and yeast. Kombucha has been around for over 2,000 years, originating around Japan. Many claims have been made about kombucha, but its primary health benefits include digestive support, increased energy, and liver detoxification.

4. Apple Cider Vinegar

    Great for controlling blood pressure, cholesterol, diabetes, and even weight loss, apple cider vinegar is a great daily addition that will bring many benefits -- including providing probiotics. Drink a small bit each day or use it as a salad dressing.

Then there is also the importance of feeding the probiotics in your system with, prebiotics.

The natural way to boost probiotics in your system is to start to feed them. So think about this: Probiotics are living organisms. If they're going live in your body, they need fuel. And the right fuel for them is fermentable fiber and prebiotics. Prebiotics are a kind of digestion resistant fiber that serves as fuel for the healthy bacteria in your gut. (187)

Prebiotics are vitally important for maintaining a healthy population of gut bacteria. If your prebiotic intake is low, your gut is going to suffer. Though that doesn't necessarily mean you need to supplement with prebiotics, though. Instead, you can get everything you need by regularly eating a variety of fruits and vegetables.

I don't see a strong need as a general guideline for most people to supplement with prebiotics. This is why we've designed the My Body Diet to be rich with prebiotic foods.

In the case of probiotics, supplementation may make more sense.

In my view, we should still start with our foods as the starting point and the main focus of nourishing our bodies, and this also goes for us having healthy guts.

With helpful bacteria less available in our food and

environment, I'm even more convinced how crucial it is to take a high-quality probiotic supplement.

This is why, in the Foundation Stack in the supplements chapter, I will walk you through the importance of probiotic supplementation.

7
WHY YOU NEED TO SLEEP TO LOSE WEIGHT

From torture to lowered brain function to overeating…

This is how lack of sleep can cause a cascade of major problems.

And why, as one of the major problems of our busy, modern-day lives, it has thrown the importance of sleep out the window.

Not sleeping enough--less than seven hours of sleep per night—can reduce and undo the benefits of dieting according to research published in the Annals of Internal Medicine.

In the study, dieters were put on different sleep schedules. When their bodies received adequate rest, half the weight they lost was from fat.

However, when they cut back on sleep, the amount of fat lost was cut in half--even though they were on the same diet. What's more, they felt significantly hungrier, were less satisfied after meals, and lacked the energy to exercise. Overall, those on a sleep-deprived diet experienced a 55 percent reduction in fat loss compared to their well-rested counterparts.

It can happen so easily, a few late nights can string together as work is busy, or you wanted to meet some friends. Or even your 7-month-old is teething and isn't sleeping well throughout the night.

Before you know it, you're in sleep debt, and when your body is sleep deprived; it suffers from "metabolic grogginess." The term was coined by University of Chicago researchers who analyzed what happened after just four days of poor sleep.

But this where I look at hacking this problem first with quality and then quantity. The National Sleep Foundation has set some solid guidelines based on their research, which have the advice of 7-9 hours of sleep for Adults (201). So, if you're not simply getting enough hours in bed, then a change in lifestyle can easily happen.

Though, helping with the quality of your sleep and ensuring you're able to get deep, restorative sleep is crucial. As I've found so many people simply lack a good night's rest, and fixing this problem has a huge carry-over effect.

As much as you want to rely on a few cups of coffee to get you through the day and back into a normal routine, your hormones that control your fat cells don't feel the same way. Within just four days of sleep deprivation, your body's ability to properly use insulin (the master storage hormone) becomes completely disrupted. In fact, the University of Chicago researchers found that insulin sensitivity dropped by more than 30 percent.

We've already walked through why dropping in insulin

sensitiveness is bad.

The hormonal cascade continues onto your hunger hormones, leptin, and ghrelin. You need to control leptin and ghrelin to successfully lose weight, but sleep deprivation makes that nearly impossible. Research published in the Journal of Clinical Endocrinology and Metabolism found that sleeping less than six hours triggers the area of your brain that increases your need for food, while also depressing leptin and stimulating ghrelin.

Each day you are learning new things, setting new memories, doing complex tasks, and all these neural networks in your brain need to organize properly. And it's not just having a lay down, or putting your feet up for a little while. It's good quality deep sleep that your brain and your body needs.

This is why, later in the book, I'm going to walk you through the Wind Down Routine, which is out first go to method to increase the quality of your sleep.

A study led by Bruce Bailey, the professor of Exercise Science at Brigham Young University, did a study where participants were assessed for body composition before and after the one-week study period.

What the researchers found was: Getting less than 6.5 hours of sleep and was linked to higher body fat. High-quality sleep was associated with lower body fat, while poor sleep correlated with higher body fat. And waking and going to sleep at the same time every day (particularly a consistent wake time) was most strongly linked with lower body fat.

The greatest effect of all was seen in the participants who woke up at the same time every morning seven days a week.

A lack of sleep can also mess with the part of the brain called the frontal lobe, which controls complex decision-making. This means you don't have the mental clarity to make good complex decisions, specifically with regards to the foods you eat--or foods you want to avoid.

This is where your brain is weakened due to sleep deprivation, you have trouble fighting the urge, and are more likely to indulge in all the wrong foods. Just another reason why you could be falling to cravings and temptations that throw you off your diet.

Not enough sleep means you're always hungry, reaching for bigger portions, and desiring every type of food that is bad for you--and you don't have the proper brain functioning to tell yourself, "No!"

Also, during sleep is when you produce a key hormone - Human Growth Hormone. One study describes Growth Hormone as have a "crucial role in consolidating and enhancing waking experience." (200)

You'll also see how we have designed the My Body Diet to also use phases of eating carbs at night to help you better sleep, along with the workouts that help produce Growth Hormone and testosterone. This is where the hard work and research has already been done for you, so all you need to do is just follow the simple plan that has all the factors working together.

8
WHY YOU CAN'T COPY MY DIET

Sitting across from me was Mary Shenouda, "The Paleo Chef," who I just had the pleasure of meeting 2 days previously. We were at Jay Ferrugia's home in LA, recording a podcast episode that completely opened my eyes to a greater way to look at food.

Mary has a very unique viewpoint and skill set where she creates incredible tasting food to nourish her clients. It was just 2-days before, when we first met, that she asked what type of music I liked.

And for me, my taste in music can range from deep house to flamenco guitar to hip-hop or to classical music depending on what I'm feeling at the time. She then went on to help me understand how she uses a person's music, home environment, blood work, and more to match what food will work for them.

This was another eye-opening experience for me, where it

showcases another reason why you can't copy just anyone's diet and expect great results from it.

One of the big issues you face is the ease and abundance of information that you are flooded with every day. And with 'internet experts' being able to spill information out at ease, I totally understand why you're feeling confused. And this is why I wanted (needed) to write this book for you.

Just like supplement companies used to 'trick' you into buying their products, you can be swept up with following a meal plan, workout, or fat-loss program that you shouldn't. By having a guy or girl totally ripped and veins running down their abs, it's easy to think that if you do what they do, then you will get the results they get.

So with supplement companies now using fitness models who are photoshopping their images to better enhance how they look, and then matching their unrealistic physique with a temptation for you to use the same supplements they use. Which often is the case, they aren't using those products at all.

So when it comes to social media and the online world flooding you with countless 'fitness experts' that are in shape themselves, they are simply regurgitating what they do and packaging that up for you to do the same thing.

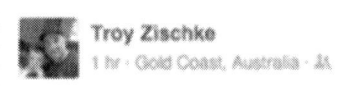

> **Troy Zischke**
> 1 hr · Gold Coast, Australia ·
>
> So 3 weeks ago before I got back on board with Chris Dufey I hopped on the scales, felt like a fat slob and weighed in at 105kgs... This morning 99kgs....WTF?!?!??,

The truth is, you can't copy my diet or plan and expect the same results.

Your mother was right. You are as unique as a snowflake, and this is why I want to give you the guiding principles, and on top of that, the knowledge so you can go through life making smarter decisions and not being confused.

It was when I was studying Functional Diagnostic Nutrition (FDN), and also interviewing the founder of FDN, Reed Davis, that it became glaringly obvious that so much of the typical advice the media and coaches are preaching these days is misleading.

Functional Diagnostic Nutrition is a type of detective work that seeks to identify the underlying causes of disease, instead of treating symptoms. Using functional lab work, we identify healing opportunities and engage each client in a health building process using the potent, proven, professional protocols in our **D.R.E.S.S. for Health Success** program. This includes **Diet, Rest, Exercise, Supplements** and **Stress Reduction**. This natural, holistic approach yields the highest level of positive clinical outcomes.

You will see much of the influence that Reed has on me flowed into being able to give you this book, the My Body Diet and the programs.

There is a huge difference between someone that can get themselves in shape and someone that can get someone else in shape. And this is why many of the 'online fitness experts' aren't giving you what you need. This is the difference between a coach that can get you the results you want and an athlete that can do it themselves. Just like in the world of sports, there is a big difference between a coach that gets the team to win and the athletes that can follow through with the plan and perform.

Robb Wolf, in his book I highly recommend 'Wired To Eat.' Shows how dramatic different peoples reaction can be to the same foods.

A large study was done by fitting the participants with a continuous glucose monitor to check their blood glucose for the duration of the study. What was so interesting from the results of the study was the difference in how people responded to foods. For example, one person would eat a banana, and they would have a great blood sugar response. Then that same person would have a terrible response to eating a cookie, which wouldn't be very surprising.

But what's so interesting is that another person would have a terrible blood sugar response to a banana, but then a great response to eating the cookie.

This is also why there are so many conflicting opinions on what you should be doing to lose weight. You've got one mob saying, "just cut all carbs out." Then another group saying, "just keep your calories and macro's in check." Then another saying, "eat paleo, and you'll lose the weight." They all work, to some degree for some people.

For me, it finally 'clicked' by learning from Chris Kresser, M.S., L.Ac who is a globally recognized leader in the fields of ancestral health, Paleo nutrition, and functional and integrative medicine.

In his book, The Paleo Cure, and with the vast amount of incredible content Chris has produced, he helps you move away from a "one perfect diet" answer. He helps you turn the popularized version of the Paleo diet into your own powerful healing tool for taking control of your health and reaching your goals.

Personally, I see it starting with a "paleo-ish" approach that first focuses on food quality, which gives you the proven set of steps to reclaim your body and health.

The answer is what is going to work for you, now and forever.

Firstly, we all react differently to foods. A study in the review journal Cell (25) shows that the blood sugar response varied from person to person, suggesting that each individual had a different reaction to carbohydrates.

Your ability to break down and absorb the foods you eat differs from person to person and because of your gut health. Even down to how well you chew your foods and start the digestion process, for example, eating carbohydrates by using the enzyme amylase that starts with your mouth. And it's your individual makeup that determines how you produce and use amylase, and this then changes the son blood sugar response to eating the same foods for each different person (25).

We then have the differences in your hormones and how

powerful these are for impacting how your body functions. We've already touched upon the factors such as sleep, meal frequency, the amount and types of foods you eat that impact metabolic hormones, and especially hunger hormones; leptin, ghrelin and neuropeptide-Y.

This then, is directly impacting whether you're craving foods, hungry and needing to eat more, and even your body's ability to burn body fat for fuel.

With the new world of epigenetics growing so rapidly at the moment, it's showing the relationship between your genetics and how your environment directly impacts how your genes respond. So it's not only your genes that you were born with that make you a unique individual, it's the environment you live in now that can change your gene expression.

Your training directly impacts your body's ability to use the foods you eat. Generally speaking, the more muscle mass you have, the higher your metabolic rate, and also the higher your insulin sensitivity. This means the amount of lean muscle you have along with the type, intensity, duration, frequency, and volume of your training impacts how your body uses the foods you eat.

Stress is another factor that will change how your body responds to the foods you eat and again your hormonal environment. We all respond differently to stress, and your mindset has a huge factor on this as well. How we each uniquely respond to stress, such as toxicity or a high-training volume. Or with lifestyle stress points, such as when you have a newborn baby, a traffic jam that has you running late for a meeting, or relationship and financial stress that we can have creep up in our modern lifestyles. All play a role in what the best foods, meals, training, and entire fat loss and lifestyle plan will work for you.

What about our lifestyles. Now that I work from my home office, I'm not a personal trainer that's on the gym floor for 12 hours a day, 6 days a week. I'm much more sedentary now, and need to use hacks like working at a standing desk to help me from falling prey to the sedentary desk job woes. **But I need to take into consideration that I may not need to eat as much food because I'm moving around a lot less. Being the geek and guinea pig I am, I track my movement with a step count each day to see how much movement I'm actually getting.**

Using the example I gave above, let's think about how having a newborn baby enter your life affects your meal and workout plan. Now having gone through this twice so far with my two daughters, it's been interesting how your body changes and what affects your body. Our first born, Arlo, is a miracle sleeper. From a very young age, she slept all the way through. From 7pm to 7am. Our youngest daughter, Sunny, is her own unique self and didn't start sleeping through the night until 9 months old.

This affected my sleep, but it affected my wife, Lauren, much more. So the increased stress from the lack of sleep building, along with the lifestyle changes that happen when a newborn comes into your life, your body is not the same as pre-baby. I'm not going to go into detail about all the changes for mothers, as that would be its own book.

And we haven't even talked about your likes, dislikes, and

personality. If your plan doesn't take this into account, you're doomed. If you love cookies and ice cream (which I do), and your meal plan strictly takes your favorite foods out, then the build-up is only going to lead up to a burst, where you binge on the foods that you're trying to avoid and cause problems both with your body and mind.

This is why I'm going to show you how to eat your favorite foods, and do it in the smart way, where you will never feel guilty because you know it's actually helping you burn fat.

The Red Pill or The Blue Pill…?

I understand that I've already given you a lot of information. We've killed off that the traditional way to losing weight by counting calories, and that the key now lies between your hormones and how you can affect your body through; the foods you eat, the way you move and exercise, the lifestyle habits you choose (or fall into), and the nutrition and supplements you can take.

This really comes down to how you can make your body work in ways that you've always wanted.

Now it's your choice. You have to make a decision: believe that you can have a better body, more confidence, less confusion, frustration, and stress following through with the rest of the guide I have for you.

Or… you can close the book and go back to what wasn't working for you before, or continue the "guessing game" to try and find the answer.

Choose wisely!

9

THE TRUTH TO LOSING WEIGHT FAST AND KEEPING IT OFF FOREVER

It all started when I was sitting in the doctor's office.

For months, I had been feeling "crappy." I was a booked out personal trainer who had a group of trainers working for me. Very rarely eating 'bad' foods or drinking alcohol and training 6 times a week.

The main problem that was really bugging me was that I couldn't get any leaner or build muscle even though I was "doing everything right." I became super strict with all my meals, I started to pull back from social events and going out for dinner. I was busting my ass in the gym every single day. Yet at the end of each week, I was barely getting leaner, and some weeks, I was getting fatter.

And this wasn't just by looking in the mirror. I was getting my body fat measurements tested each week to make sure I was measuring everything that I needed to. And in all honesty, life started to suck.

And then, he laughed.

The doctor, who is a great functional medicine doctor in Sydney actually laughed when he saw the lab results that had come in. My testosterone was that of an old man's. Even though I was about 12% body fat and had a decent level of muscle mass on me, on the inside, I was weak, unhealthy, and underperforming.

And I was 22 years old.

Having just bought my first home, being busy, and stressed with running the personal training business, being indoors for most of the day for 6 days a week training and consulting clients stopping me from getting out in the sun. All of this was cooking an unhealthy concoction that was being led by a diet that was low in calories, low in carbs, and doubled up with a super high amount of training.

I walked out of the doctor's office angry. I was doing everything I was told to do from the gurus, and this was now the result I was in.

This is why you should ask yourself; "Why am I stuck with the same results, no matter what I do to change my body?"

The first answer to this is the missing information. It was a 10-minute walk from the doctor's office; up Manly beach to my home in Queenscliff, and that was exactly what my answer was. I didn't have the right information, as everything I was doing, clearly, wasn't working.

This step that I had to take is the same step that you should take right now. All the right information is in this book for you. And, as you're going to see in the coming chapters, we are going to clean your plate of the lies and mistruths that have held you back. And then I'm going to give you the focus you need, with the simple to follow plan so that you have the life-changing experience that I had, and, gratefully, have watched so many others have.

And this may be the hardest part for you. It's that you must let go of past beliefs and the biases that you currently hold. For me, it took a slap to the face truth from lab results showing that my hormones and body were being crippled along with my physique not getting leaner, even though I was sacrificing my social life.

Especially when it comes to nutrition, it's amazing how everyone has their opinion and their beliefs. You try telling a vegan to go eat some beef, and you'll probably be slapped. You tell a 'low-carber' to chill out and eat a packet of cookies with you, and they'll laugh at you. The strong biases that are held are the main problems holding so many people back. The health and fitness industry has turned into people wanting, not to debate and progress as a whole, but to prove someone wrong and 'one up' them to win.

That's why there was a recurring theme, in preparing to write this book for you, and with the previous 11 years of reviewing as much diet and fitness information as possible. This theme was also present in the wins and fails for myself and clients, the courses, certifications, books, mentors, and consultations.

This is the theme of what it really took to bring about jaw-dropping results. And that's being able to burn off the unwanted fat, keep it off, enjoy the process, and happily get on with life is a hell of a lot easier than so many make it out to be. The health and weight industry is fueled by making it hard, confusing, and setting you up for dependence on all the 'secrets' that each program tries to lure you with.

And that's why all the clients' and your success isn't about doing a workout or eating certain foods. It starts with something much tougher. And that is, that you now need to reject most of what people believe to be true when it comes to weight loss.

That's why, from this chapter, there are only two things you need to follow. To make this a realistic, easy to stick to plan. And one that gets you into the best shape of your life, and loving your life at the same time.

1. Learn the truth - You're going to find out how your body works, and why so many factors such as; your sleep, the foods you choose, the way you move your body, what nutrients you could be lacking, how your daily stress impacts you, and how and what hormones are affected by all the previous points, and how this ultimately has you looking, feeling, and functioning the way you want.

After traveling the world and going to see the top coaches and experts, I learned one of the most important points from Christian Maurice who is a highly sort after coach who is known for getting some of the most famous actors in shape for their roles.

> "An educated client is an adherent client."

This is exactly what I wrote down after he said it, sitting in his office in Montreal, Canada. It's something that I've taken to heart throughout my career, and it's one reason why I've had the success so far in transforming bodies.

This is what I'm doing with you right now. You need to "buy in" on what this book and plan have for you. You, having this book in your hands and reading it, is a very serious thing to me. And I'm treating you like a private client because I want you to get the best results possible.

2. Follow the plan - Then it's putting everything to use and having the simple to follow plan go to work for you. I understand that change is hard, and you would rather jump on the couch to watch a movie with a tub of Ben and Jerrys.

   But what I'm here to say, is that there will be time for that. Though you are also going to need to do your workouts and make the changes needed so you are feeding your body the foods that will turn you into a fat burning machine. And then, you can dive headfirst into your favorite foods and know it's helping you shape the body you want.

One of the world's top, influential minds that I've been thankful to interview and learn from multiple times is Vince Del Monte. And from our very first conversation, and each interview thereafter, the same theme has come up, "A good coach makes plans realistic for people."

And this is one reason why Vince can help transform thousands of bodies, as the plans are made for the everyday you and me to be able to follow. The aim here is progression, not perfection. And why, if you've constantly failed to lose weight and transform your body before, it can be because the plan was simply not made to suit you.

We now need to tackle the lies and mistruths that have been holding you back. And at the same time, break away and take one of the most important steps that is going to transform your body.

10
"YOU NEED TO EAT EVERY 2-HOURS TO 'STOKE YOUR METABOLISM.'"

We've all heard it before, and I was one of those dudes that was carrying around every meal in a Tupperware container. Because, god forbid, if I didn't eat within 2-3 hours of my last meal, my metabolism was going to drop, and I could lose precious muscle.

You need to reject the belief that you need to eat frequently to stoke your metabolism. Not only is it just utterly inconvenient when trying to live a life, it's not proven by science to work.

Better yet, by being smarter with when you time your meals, you can increase your body's ability to burn body fat and have a host of health benefits, all of which I'll show you very soon.

Let me introduce you to Adam as we first met in a mid-afternoon day in a hot, dry, Bali gym.

For the past 3 years now, I've had the luxury of working from home and choosing the design of how I want my days to go. The time that I work out for myself is usually around 2pm, and I've always found it fascinating the interesting people I bump into who also train at this time. They are also usually people who have broken the typical 9-5 work mold and have interesting stories.

I'll admit, that when I am training, I'm not the most outgoing and interactive type of guy. I'm a get in, get out, and get the job done person. But I had noticed this guy training at the same time as myself a few times and could tell he knew what he was doing when it came to training properly. So I introduced myself, and that's when Adam and I began our friendship.

He is a professional poker player and had a keen interest in health and fitness. I invited him to come and train with me, and I would happily share my training programs and nutrition guidelines for him to use. He gratefully accepted, and instantly, I could tell he was serious about making a big change for himself.

For so long, he had been training hard and "doing everything right." But was still struggling with slow progress, and not being able to build the muscle or get lean. The plans that I gave him are exactly what I am giving you here with this book and with the bonuses.

He was perplexed as to why so much of what I was recommending was flying in the face of so much of the mainstream advice he had been reading and learning. This was when I could easily explain how much simpler a meal plan can be, and why our training sessions were so different to what he had done before.

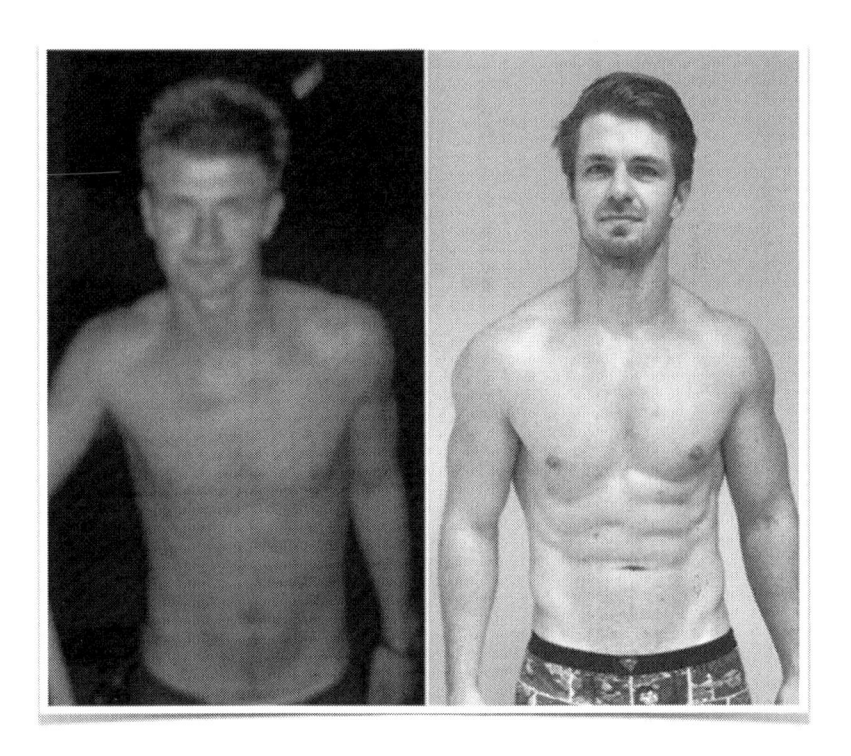

Now you can see the transformation that he's been able to create for himself. But what I enjoy so much out of this, is how easily he has been able to make it happen. By actually following an eating window of 6-8 hours of feeding each day. Understanding when and how much he can happily enjoy starchy carbs and by eating more than he was before, he is now able to stay lean year round.

Where this myth probably came from was the fact that digesting a meal raises metabolism, and this is known as the Thermic Effect of Food. This is simply the metabolic process of where your body has to use energy to break down food to then digest the energy. A meta-analysis done on eating frequency found no difference in 24-hour energy expenditure from whether you nibbled multiple meals through the day or gorged all your food at once, assuming you're eating the same quantity of food (26). This shows us pretty clearly that eating 6 meals a day does not help you burn more fat.

I also expect that because diet dogma can come from people simply copying and regurgitating what someone else is doing, that following the typical bodybuilder diet has slid its way into the fat-loss diet belief. If you have a bodybuilder who is needing to eat 4,000 to 6,000 calories a day, there is no way he or she can comfortably eat that amount of food in just a few meals. So they would need to eat more frequency to comfortably digest their food throughout the day.

That's why, with the plan I will lay out for you, we take a more realistic approach, and find the use of having a larger gap between meals throughout the week. What you will learn is a method of Intermittent Fasting can have a great effect in turning you into a fat burning machine.

This is where we can inject some 'common sense' and use a window of time each day that you can happily choose how many meals you want to eat in that window.

For example, you could have a 12-hour eating window. So if your last meal of the day is at 8pm, then your first meal of the day is at 8am. And you can just space your meals out to whatever suits you. Though why we give guidelines to start, is so that it makes it easier for you to find what suits your metabolism and your lifestyle together.

We know that if you're eating at the same times each day, you're going to become hungry at those times. So when making changes to your meal timing and frequency, we want to avoid you having hunger pangs due to the fact that you've been eating at the same time of the day for a long time.

You get to be able to have a plan that's backed by science, but also have it easily fit in with your lifestyle, so there's no pressure.

11
"BREAKFAST IS THE MOST IMPORTANT MEAL OF THE DAY"

"Breakfast is the most important meal of the day"… Sound familiar?

It sure does to me, because this is exactly what used to fly out of my mouth when coaching my clients years ago. This is one of the foundational pieces of weight loss advice that comes from trainers to doctors.

The only problem though is that it's wrong!

There is no 'special meal,' and you'll soon see, as I walk you through the My Body Diet, that breakfast can be pushed back a few hours to help you burn fat and build muscle.

It's not that I don't like breakfast. It's just that when you lengthen the window you're eating each day and double up eating the wrong foods for breakfast, you can be switching off your fat burning metabolism and setting yourself up to be hungrier throughout the day.

Observational studies consistently show that breakfast skippers are more likely to be obese than people who eat breakfast (27). But this is where correlation doesn't mean causation. It does not prove that breakfast helps you lose weight. It's just that it's associated with a lower risk of obesity. It's just like the science that shows a relationship between flossing and better heart health. It's likely that it's not the flossing that causes better heart health, it's that people that floss take better care of their health, and it's just a correlation.

I did come upon a study of 309 (49) overweight and obese but otherwise healthy adults in two random groups where the researchers specifically wanted to find out whether eating or not eating breakfast had any impact on weight loss. After 16 weeks, the researchers found no difference in weight loss between the groups. In essence, it didn't matter if they ate breakfast or not.

In one study in teenage girls, a high-protein breakfast significantly reduced cravings (82).

Again, this is where we tailor the plan to suit you. Some people feel great having breakfast, and other people opt to eat later in the day. This is where you can have flexibility and not fall prey to the "there's only one way to eat" idea. This is why, though, most diets are flawed. They set you up with psychological barriers that make it harder for you to live a real life and abide by their rules.

You're soon going to learn about having a compressed eating window, also known as Intermittent fasting. This not only debunks the previous myth of "eat small frequent meals to stoke your metabolism," it can also set you up to have profound health benefits along with helping you burn off the stubborn fat.

As an author, I try my best to push personal bias out of the way. And I have found that eating between 12 midday to 8pm at night, I've been able to stay much leaner, much easier throughout the year. I'm not worrying or even thinking about food, as hunger is not a problem, and my mental focus is much better.

This is why in the 5-Steps to Losing Weight I'm going to walk you through some simple, yet powerful strategies that you can mold to fit your likes and lifestyle to see the effects on your own body.

12
"YOU SHOULD EAT CARBS AT THE START OF THE DAY"

Then there is the importance of eating the right foods and looking at how you can easily use 'nutrient timing' to accelerate your weight loss. Avoiding carbs in the morning actually goes against the current mainstream thinking whereby people assume it is best to eat carbs in the morning when you are more 'insulin sensitive.' While this is a shady gray area of belief - the 'pro' breakfast carb crowd say that you are more insulin sensitive in the morning and therefore will tolerate carbs better - this does not necessarily mean you should eat carbs in the morning though.

Let me take you back to 2009 when I first walked into a seminar with Charles Poliquin. I would have walked out with an entire exercise book of notes, and quickly went to work in trying everything out. On the very next morning, I remember testing out the "meat and nut breakfast."

The basics of this are that you are to start the day with a protein and fat-rich meal that will positively influence your brain neurotransmitters and stabilize blood sugar and energy levels for the day to come. One of Poliquin's favorite teaching axioms is "The first thing you put in your mouth in the morning…provided it is food…dictates all neurotransmitters for the whole day." For myself, I immediately noticed a difference that first day, so I quickly got onto sharing this with all my clients.

And the reports coming back were astounding. In all my years of coaching, I've only had one female client that thrived on a carb-heavy meal to start the day. This isn't to say that you cut all carbs out of your first meal of every day, it's that we can be smarter and be a detective to find out what truly works for you in setting up your meal plan.

John Kiefer also points out in "Carb Backloading," that you are better off not raising insulin at all in the first part of the day; rather, extending the natural fat burning (fasted) state after sleeping.

Let's use right now as an example. As I'm writing this for you, it's 9am in the morning. I've been up for about 3 hours so far, and I haven't eaten anything. For roughly the past 2 years, I've been experimenting with Intermittent Fasting and timing of nutrients. In a very simple sense, I've been eating breakfast a little later (which I'll talk more on soon) and eating my carbs at the end of the day. This is using metabolic flexibility to my favor as the first half of my day is focused on being in a fat burning state.

So while I do the majority of my work (and can have my brain optimally working) and not have to be worried about food or hunger as I get my work done, I also am in a better 'fat burning' state. You'll also discover soon that by not eating as soon as you awake you can have your cellular clean up called 'autophagy' being maximized to help your natural detox systems.

The better you can manage your insulin, and also help promote greater Growth Hormone, the better your body can burn body fat for fuel.

I know, I know…

Eating meat and nuts for breakfast might seem a little odd for you, and you'd rather not cook up a steak for your first meal. This is perfectly fine, and it's why in the My Body Diet we can use a variety of different meats along with a smoothie to nourish you with ample protein, fats, and nutrients.

13

"EAT LOW CARBS TO LOSE THE WEIGHT."

This one is my favorites… Because it was when I finally broke free from 'low-carb life,' I not only started getting leaner and building muscle, I started enjoying the whole process, as well as having the pleasure of being able to live life and not be constantly stressed about every next meal.

We've covered a lot already, especially how your food, movement, and lifestyle impact your hormones and how they are affecting how you look, feel, and function day to day. And that's why it's important for you to understand what really matters when it comes to getting in shape. There are usually two sides to this argument, and the truth is, the answer will usually fall somewhere in the middle.

On one side of the pendulum we have the 'low carbers,' and

even now, the strong surge for ketogenic diets. With their main argument being that if you keep insulin in check, then your body is going to be able to burn fat and not easily gain fat. And on the other side of the pendulum, we have the "calories is a calorie" crowd who want to just keep your total calorie intake under your overall expenditure and you'll lose weight.

Now we've already touched on why both of these aren't entirely true. But we need to delve into what I believe is needed, and that's the smart carb approach. Being able to nourish yourself with foods that give your body what it needs, and have you happily eating those foods, so you're not feeling restricted.

As the low-carb claim goes; Insulin "makes you fat," and carbohydrates spike insulin. Therefore, "carbohydrates make you fat." If you just eat fewer carbs, your insulin is lower and you will lose all the weight. It's a nice simple formula, but it's just not entirely true.

This is why I've showcased and interviewed Mike T Nelson with much of the focus on 'Metabolic Flexibility.'

> Metabolic flexibility is the ability to switch from one fuel source to the next. Due to possible discontinuities in both the supply and demand for energy, humans need a clear capacity to use fats and carbohydrate fuels and transition between them.
> What you want to be able to have happen, is to switch from one fuel source to the next. And where Metabolic Inflexibility is where you have the limited ability to switch from one fuel source to the next. In a healthy state with normal insulin metabolism, humans can

effectively switch from a primarily fat metabolism to a carbohydrate metabolism, and vice versa.

And what is going to work for you, is not going to work for someone else. That's why you're going to find that the first phase I take you through with the My Body Diet is the 14-Day Metabolic Switch.

This is bringing your carbohydrate intake down so we can get your body to efficiently and effectively be able to use carbs later. Combine this together with smarter workouts, and you're turning your body into a fat burning machine (you become more metabolically flexible).

The big problem that comes about when you're told to just "eat fewer carbs" is that it's so individual. We've already covered that variables, such as how often your training, the type of workouts you're doing, the level of muscle mass you have, stress management, insulin sensitivity, how well you sleep, and a host of other factors come into play to determine how well your body can handle carbohydrates.

Not all carbs are created equal, and saying that "carbs are bad" is like vilifying all fats and not seeing the difference between Omega-3 fats and trans fats. Having deep-fried potato chips that are cooked in corn oil and swimming in dipping sauce is not the same as eating a baked potato. There's also the demonizing of fruit because of fructose.

Fructose has been bashed because it's clearly shown that high fructose corn syrup is a nasty substance for the human body and something found in a lot of processed foods, such as cakes, cookies, breakfast cereals, nutrition bars. Even worse, is that the labeling for high fructose corn syrup can legally be written as maize syrup, glucose syrup, tapioca syrup, and more. All of which make it harder for, you the consumer, to dodge the nasty products.

The big takeaway point is that there is a huge difference between high fructose corn syrup and eating an apple that has fructose in it. One of the big reasons is the amount of fructose that is in the apple is far less. The apple is in its whole form which means it comes with the fiber, water, and nutrients that are good for you. And the actual chemical difference of high fructose corn syrup and fructose found in whole fruit is different.

> One of the reasons why I designed the My Body Diet is to have you going through a simple cycle of what fuels your body is burning. This is why in the beginning phase, while your body is still burning sugar as its primary fuel, we focus your food choices to have you regain metabolic flexibility to burn fat.
> Then we can easily double, triple or quadruple your carbohydrate intake because the metabolic "magic" actually happens during the refeeding phase. Dr. Steve Gundry was one of the experts that speaks to this with his books, The Diet Evolution and The Plant Paradox.

No longer do I want you to just see things in black and white. As so many health gurus set you up for failure by seeing foods as simply 'good' and 'bad.' Healthy is a relative term, and it's about what is going to work for you, so you are in the body you want, functioning and performing at the level you want each day and being able to enjoy the process.

One of the reasons low-carb diets work so well is that they reduce appetite. They make people eat fewer calories automatically, so there is no need for calorie counting or portion control (14, 29). This is where we can combine what is going to optimize your important metabolic hormones like insulin, but also have you feeling satisfied from each meal and naturally having calories under control without ever having to count them.

Research has shown that some people's bodies deal better with large amounts of dietary fat than others, responding with positive metabolic changes like an increase in resting energy expenditure and fat oxidation to maintain energy balance, and better appetite control. (30)

In all honesty, it was first reading Tim Ferriss' 'The 4-Hour Body' and his work on the Slow Carb Diet that finally had it 'click' for me.

For years, I was trying to make sense of all the information and research into how to best structure diets and training for fat loss. It's been applying and experimenting with variations of the Slow Carb Diet along with the knowledge of the other top experts and leaders that has led to the My Body Diet.

Technically they are very similar, though you will find that I want to give you some starting principles that can help kickstart your results, and set you up for long-term success. As you will find the success that comes from the Slow Carb Diet is the sheer simplicity.

To make this super simple, there is no need to dive deeply into the science. You do need to understand the basics of what the different foods you can put in your mouth do to your body. But this is also why I'm going to walk you through the My Body Diet, so you know what foods to eat, when to eat, and how much of them to eat. But also, you will be able to easily shop, prepare, and cook your foods as well, without having to read every label, get confused on what the best choices are, and waste hours each week when you just have to follow the simple guidelines I'm going to give you.

14

"CARDIO IS THE BEST WAY TO LOSE WEIGHT"

Running is one of the most popular ways to exercise to lose weight. And why I wanted to write this entire book for you was to clear out the mistruths, and give you the simple to follow guide to get the best results while enjoying your life.

And there's a good chance that if you're like me, you've slogged it out with hours of cardio before. And especially when it comes to 'pounding the pavement' and going out for long runs, this is NOT the effective fat-loss strategy you should be using.

Now before we delve into why and what else you can be doing to get far greater results, I want to cover 'what you enjoy.' As so many fitness gurus and trainers are just jumping on one fad after another. Lately, it's that High-Intensity Interval Training (HIIT) is the best thing for fat loss. Now HIIT training is very effective, and I will show you how you can use it as a part of your program, but what if you just don't enjoy it?

You also have on the other side of the pendulum, the long duration cardio, which can also be done while in a fasted state.

Why I'm not a fan of having my main focus of going out for a run being lose weight is because the belief that is still ingrained in so much of the mainstream weight loss advice is that you just need to burn calories. And going for a 45 or even 60-minute run is going to burn calories and also be in the "fat burning zone." This is the heart rate zone, where you have a majority of your fuel being used as fat.

The problem with this is that it's only looking at the small window of time that you are training. It doesn't look at the other 23 hours of the day, and that's where EPOC (excess post-exercise oxygen consumption) is far more efficient by using Metabolic Resistance and Metabolic Conditioning training.

Brad Schoenfeld put so well when he said, "It's short-sighted to look at how much fat is burned during a radio session… Fat burning must be considered over the course of days, not on an hour to hour basis."

It's also why we designed the training so that we can take advantage of having lower insulin levels and lower glycogen, along with elevated cortisol so that there can be greater fat oxidization.

So rather than going out and pounding the pavement with long runs, endless spin classes, and tireless cardio sessions, I'll show you how we start with Metabolic Resistance Training to give you the best bang for your buck in your workouts.

There's also the hybrid training that we use with the My Body

Diet, and that is Metabolic Conditioning training (Met Con). This is the use of resistance training to bring about a different effect, that along with your Metabolic Resistance Training, is a powerful tool for effective fat loss.

Then there is the 'yin' style of exercise, and for me, I really enjoy walking. I walk for at least 30 minutes every day as well as surfing and doing some yoga whenever I can fit it in. Walking is one of the most underrated forms of movement, and if you would see me going for my walks, you would barely classify it as exercise. It's more of a gentle walk as I'm usually listening to an audio book, podcast, or thinking to myself making notes on my phone.

You now know that working with greater intensity and using a lot of muscle can deplete your immediate energy stores. Depleting blood glucose, stored glycogen, intramuscular fat, and free fatty acids through high-intensity work means the body must then obtain energy from other sources. This is where you force it to use your body fat in two ways.

But then there is the hormonal factor that can come with overdoing the cardio. Along with cognitive and brain function decline, lowered immune function, and damaged reproductive health excess cortisol promotes fat storage and muscle loss. This can happen because cortisol can lower testosterone, and excess cardio has been shown to increase cortisol levels.

This is where we come to the difference between "it doesn't work" and "it doesn't work as well." As there are a lot of fitness professionals jumping up and down and saying cardio is causing massive health problems and even weight gain. This, again, is the pendulum being swung too far the other way. And there are many great benefits of doing cardio, especially if you enjoy it as well.

If you enjoy Zumba classes, then I want you doing Zumba classes. It might not be 'ideal' for fat loss, but it's far better than trying to do something that you don't enjoy and eventually give up. But this is where I am writing this for you to combine the fastest path to fat loss and you getting the body you want, along with what's realistic and is going to work in a day to day scenario for you enjoying life.

15

"DON'T WORRY ABOUT SUPPLEMENTS, THEY ARE A WASTE OF MONEY"

There are two questions I get asked back to back on a weekly basis. "Do I need nutritional supplements if I'm eating a healthy diet?" and "what should I be taking?"

And there's no doubt that you're probably feeling utterly confused when it comes to trying to find answers to these two questions. We've all seen the ridiculous claims certain supplement companies are making, and even worse is the number of supplement companies that have now been heavily fined or put out of business for their shady practices. Leading up to writing this chapter, I interviewed Ryan Munsey, who works with Natural Stacks. Ryan is someone who I've only recently been introduced to, but have a deep respect for the work he is doing along with Natural Stacks for their ethical and high-quality work with the supplements they make.

For myself, I had to scratch my own itch. As for years, I was spending hundreds of dollars every month on supplements and had no idea what was working and what was not. This was when I started my journey of diving into learning about what the body needs and how to best give it. This is what also got me to start My Body Blends and to create the supplements that I ultimately wanted. Our first product, Superfood Blend, was a product myself, my wife, and daughter, Arlo (who was two and a half at the time) were taking on a daily basis.

I quickly learned, in an ideal world, we wouldn't need supplements. But without modern lifestyle, the poor quality of food, and our daily exposure to stress and toxins, we need to give our bodies the raw ingredients needed so our bodies can thrive.

And this is where there is a difference between the food you were eating 20 to 30 years ago and the foods you are eating today. And the main culprit of this disturbing difference is what is happening with soil depletion. Modern agricultural practices have stripped the soil of nutrients, and therefore, the food that is grown today is depleted and lackluster with the nutrients we need for our bodies to thrive.

Donald David and his team of researchers from the University of Texas at Austin's Department of Chemistry and Biochemistry was published in December 2004 in the Journal of the American College of Nutrition found "reliable declines" in key nutrients. "Efforts to breed new varieties of crops that provide greater yield, pest resistance, and climate adaptability have allowed crops to grow bigger and more rapidly," reported Davis, "but their ability to manufacture or uptake nutrients has not kept pace with their rapid growth."

Simply, the methods which are being used to grow bigger, more of, even growing produce for a different taste and color, and pest resistance is harming the quality of our nutrition. In addition, most plants are not harvested fresh. They sit on trucks, shelves, and counters for weeks before being eaten. Over time, the nutrient content of these plants decreases. When plants contain fewer nutrients, the animals that eat these plants are also malnourished. A study published in the Journal of Nutrition and Health found copper levels in the UK have dropped by 90% in dairy, 55% in meat, and 76% in vegetables.

Crops are raised in soil where nutrients have been depleted. Plants are treated with pesticides and other chemicals, so they no longer have to fight to live, which further diminishes their nutrient levels and their phytonutrient content (not to mention the toxic exposure you receive from such chemicals). Animals are cooped up in pens or giant feedlots instead of roaming free eating the nutrient-rich wild grains and grasses they once consumed. Since cows' stomachs are adapted to grass instead of corn, they must take antibiotics to prevent them from ill health.

There is also the problem that a 'low-calorie diet is a low nutrient diet.' When following the guide we give you with the My

Body Diet, you are focusing on nutrient-rich foods. Though I have no doubt that the "eat less, to lose more weight" belief is not going to suddenly stop with my publishing this book, my hopes are that it will make a dent. However, I know that I will continue to publish more books, resources, videos, interviews, and help so people will make smarter decisions for their physique and health. There is also the IIFYM 'If It Fits Your Macro's' that, unfortunately, like many diet beliefs, have been prostituted and twisted.

The whole 'flexible dieting' approach is to empower each of us to have a choice of the foods we eat and how we eat them. Instead, many people are 'missing the forest for the trees' in our flexible approach, and trying to maximize how many poor-quality foods they can eat and justify it with simply "fitting in with their macronutrient goals."

The reason why a 'macronutrient counting' method does NOT work for the vast majority is that the structure and the need to be constantly calculating your food intake is not possible for so many people. And it's the IIFYM advocates that are the ones that can easily track their food intake each day. Now this is perfectly fine. If a plan is working for you, fantastic. Keep using the plan.

Coming from the physique model and bodybuilding world, I and countless others, who because of the constant weighing, counting, measuring, and therefore, thinking and stressing on food open the gates to eating disorders.

This is why I wrote this book for the many, many people that have not been able to lose weight with these types of diets.

Next, we also need to deal with the toxic environment we

simply cannot escape. And rather than crying about it, we can be simply smarter about what we need to do to win the battle against toxins. And as a part of the natural detox process, your body needs certain nutrients to rid it of these harmful chemicals, which again, places a bigger burden on the nutritional needs of your body.

Finally, we also have the need to absorb the foods we eat. And with gut health being a major problem for so many, we need to face the facts that your body might not be soaking up the nutrients from the foods you eat.

Simply put, all of us are exposed to hazardous toxins and chemicals that poison our bodies, we live with too much stress, we don't sleep enough, we don't exercise enough, and we are inflamed making the nutritional demands on our bodies even heavier.

Even in the words of Dr. Mark Hyman; "In today's world, everyone needs a basic multivitamin and mineral supplement. The research is overwhelming on this point (31). My own experience as a practitioner corresponds to what the research tells us. I have tested for vitamin and nutrient deficiencies in thousands of patients and found that by correcting them people feel better, improve their mood, mental sharpness, memory and ability to focus, as well as have more energy, resolve chronic health complaints or conditions and even lose weight. Taking supplements also helps prevent disease."

The problem I know you face (and it's why I literally scratched my own itch and had to start making the products myself) is that you're probably asking, "what products can I trust and are going to work?" Be aware that all brands are not created equally. Quality is up to the manufacturer because of limited regulations regarding manufacturing. Certain companies are more careful about quality, sourcing of raw materials, consistency of dose from batch to batch, the use of active forms of nutrients, not using fillers, additives, colorings, etc. When choosing supplements, it is important that you choose quality products.

16

WHY YOUR WILLPOWER IS FAILING YOU

This is one topic that has consumed me for a long time, and because I know how horrible you can be feeling when you have yet again failed at sticking to your diet. You're motivated and driven, yet even with your best intentions, 'stuff' happens, and you find yourself having eaten something you know you shouldn't have.

The truth is, you did not fail in the diet. The diet failed you. The majority of weight loss programs are set for you to fail. They are not designed with either the true understanding of how the body works or the integration of the mind, they also fail to take into account that we're living a modern-day life.

This is why I want you to introduce you to @just_a_girl_into_fitness.

You see on the right-hand side of this picture that this is the bubbly personality, and is the person who walked through the gym doors when I was a personal trainer in Dubai. I had the pleasure of coaching @just_a_girl_into_fitness, and when she said, "Chris helped me to stop eating my feelings."

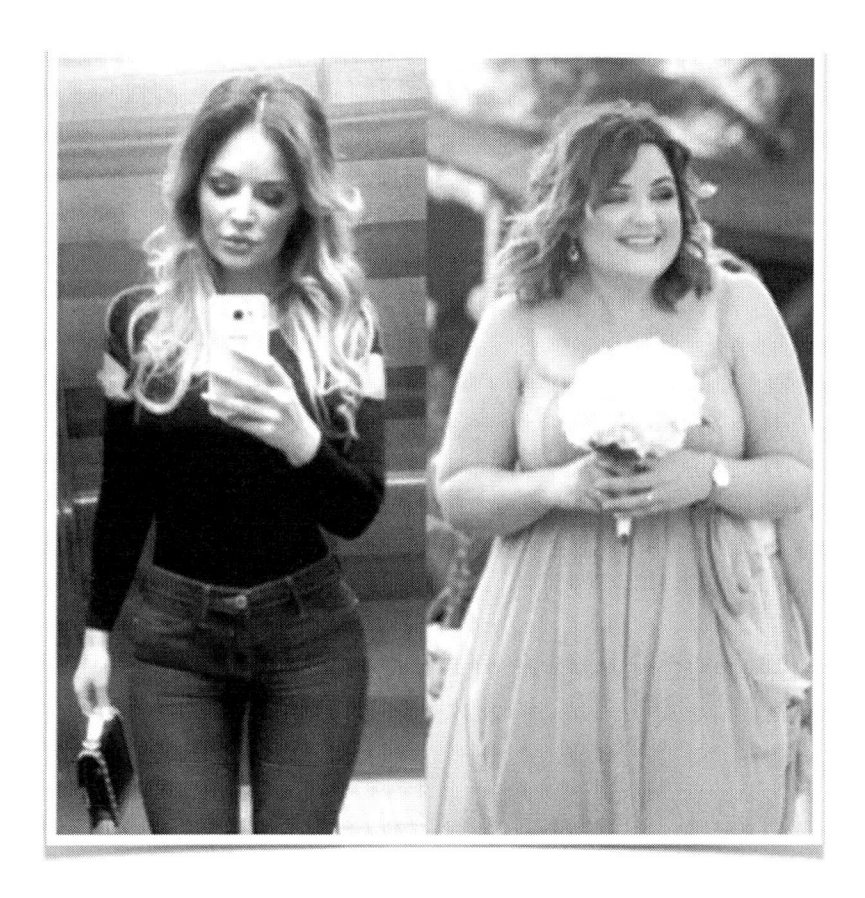

It was one of the best compliments as a coach I have received. And this really struck a deep chord within me. Because this was the exact problem I had battled with for so long.

When the diet or weight loss program you're trying to follow is telling you that you are the problem if you can't stick with the plan, it can be a soul sucking and desperate situation. You're left in a constant spiral of having to gain motivation and picking yourself up only to find yourself falling back off and battling with the plan.

As you can see now, she has dramatically transformed her body. But it's not the physical transformation that most impresses me. It's the total self-transformation that happened. The mind and the body need to change together.

When you are trying to get through each day gritting your teeth and exerting self-discipline to force yourself to follow through with the plan at hand, you're ultimately going to fail. And it's because it has been shown that willpower is like a battery. You will wear it down throughout the day, and it will ultimately lead to the exhaustion of emotions, with your impulses and cravings taking over.

On the other hand, I'm not going to pat you on the back and so it's all ok, and the weight you want to lose can just fall off without any effort or work from you. You have to take responsibility for yourself and the results you get in every area of life.

This was famously shown in the 'marshmallow test' that was performed at Stanford University. It was a series of studies on delayed gratification by psychologist Walter Mischel. What happened was a child was offered either a marshmallow or a cookie. And the scientist offering the treat would say that they are going to leave the room, and if they didn't eat it while they were gone, they would get a second treat upon their return. (32)

So the child was offered one small reward immediately or two small rewards if they waited a short period of time; testing if they could use delayed gratification. In the follow-up studies, the researchers found that the children that were able to have delayed gratification and therefore not eat the treat and wait to get the greater reward tended to have better life outcomes.

The researchers followed each child for more than 40 years, and over and over again, the group who had waited patiently for the second marshmallow succeeded in whatever capacity they were measuring. In other words, this series of experiments proved that the ability to delay gratification was critical for success in life.

I want to share this with you because you're able to see this play out everywhere. If you delay gratification and don't watch TV and do your homework instead, you'll get better grades. If you delay gratification and not procrastinate, but instead, get the marketing or client work done, your business will flourish.

And the same applies to this very book. If you don't eat the foods you know you shouldn't and delay gratification, you can lose the weight. Success usually comes down to choosing the pain of discipline over the ease of distraction. And that's exactly what delayed gratification is all about.

There are two sides to this coin, though. You cannot just grit your teeth and avoid all the foods you want, and completely deny yourself with the things you want. It would be great if every spare second between working on my businesses and having time with my family, I was studying and learning. And trust me, I've gone through times where I tried. Literally reading 2-3 hours a day and listening to audio books or interviews for another 2-3 hours whenever I was walking, cooking, or had time in between tasks, I was trying to fill my brain with information. But the truth is, you need to have a release valve every now and then and have what can be called balance.

This is the same as your food. If you think you can be a robot and just only eat chicken and broccoli for the rest of your life to be in a lean and muscular body, you're kidding yourself. One reason I know this, is because I've tried to do this for a very long time, and I know many other competitive physique athletes who have as well. And this is where understanding you as a human being on both a psychological and physiological aspect, we now know that it's a very good thing to still enjoy your cookies and ice cream (that's what I love, you can insert your own favorite foods).

Accepting the human trait that there is the struggle of self-discipline, I want to set you up for automatic success by giving you the easy to follow plan that doesn't build-up these internal struggles that can often lead to explosions (like eating an entire pint of Ben and Jerry's and a bag of peanut M&Ms), or having another excuse to skip the gym for the third day in a row. The plan will also help you to build your 'self-discipline muscle,' so that you can make the decisions, when needed, to bring about the success you want and in any area of your life.

Then there is the physiological aspect that comes into play here, and that is; dopamine.

An example of this is when the thought of eating the Ben and Jerry's ice cream comes flooding into your mind with a thought like "wouldn't that be nice," you can have a surge of dopamine in the brain that then has you fixated on that thought, and the pleasure you're going to get from it (33).

What really turns this into a shit storm is that you can have an insulin spike in anticipation of the food, which therefore, lowers your blood sugar levels and makes you crave the ice cream even more (34). And then, to make matters even worse, when dopamine is released, it also triggers the release of stress hormones which can make you feel anxious (35). So this is why it suddenly becomes more important to you, and why you want it even more.

So imagine strolling down through the supermarket to get some quick food after a long day at work. You're tired, a little stressed, already hungry, and you've used up your willpower through the day making the right food decisions, getting your workout done in the morning, and making the right decisions at work. Then the stroll past the ice cream section has just turned into a fat-gaining storm in a matter of seconds.

Do you remember the Pringles advert; "Once you pop, you can't stop?"

They were correct! They designed the food to be highly palatable and to play on the brain in the way that you're are just wanting to keep eating them.

This is why I want to show you how to tackle this problem and succeed by having the plan and tools that will help you from falling prey to this ever so common problem.

17

THE TRUTH OF 'DETOX' FOR FAT LOSS

If you're feeling sluggish with low energy…

If you're having trouble losing weight and keeping it off…

If you want to quickly kickstart your system so you can start looking, feeling, and performing better each day…

You might find yourself looking into how a 'detox' can be the answer.

From water cleanses to juice fasts, to shakes that promise more energy and fast weight loss. It's easy to be swept up in the hype.

The problem with so many of these quick detoxes is that they don't work, and they can often make you even more toxic than when you started. This is why I have spent so much time with, and have showcased Dr. Bob Rakowski multiple times on the Limitless Body Podcast.

The Truth of 'Detox' For Fat Loss

It was over 6 years ago now that I was putting myself through a strict training and nutrition plan in preparation for a photoshoot. I was "doing everything right" and sticking to the plan 100%. But I hit a plateau.

And after training harder and for longer, and cutting my food down even further, my fat loss had still stalled and not budged. It had become an all-consuming worry and frustration as to why nothing was working. It was soon after that, I discovered Dr. Bob Rakowski and his teaching and methods on how to help the body go throughputs natural detox process.

So I dove in head first and decided to do a 7-day plan that had further 7 days after slowly re-introducing foods back into my diet. This plan has now been modified over the years with constant fine tuning to what we now use with our members today, ones that have been able to drastically break through fat-loss plateaus, but even more importantly, improve health markers and their sense of vitality and energy for day to day living.

With my first encounter of going through what we call a "nutritional cleanse," I was able to get leaner than I ever had, and my wife, Lauren, and I conceived our first child. Honestly, this is not a magic potion or formula. You're going to find out in this chapter what it's all about, and how you can add this to your day to day living.

Now, we have to be honest.

If you're battling with hunger, you're overeating, and struggling to lose weight, the most common causes is that you're under-eating, eating the 'wrong' types of foods, and/or over exercising. This is also why we focus on the key pillars of your health, which are sleep, stress, lifestyle, and giving you the emotional support to be able to make the changes that give you the body, mind, and life you want.

But to not include the insights into how you can help your body detox and lower your toxic burden would make this book incomplete for you. This is also why I have showcased the Magnificent 7 that Dr. Bob Rokawski has created. And you will see that much of what this book covers (and programs entail for members) includes exactly what Dr. Bob has so elegantly put together:

The Magnificent 7.

Eat Right: "You are what you eat." We need to eat foods that build our bodies up and avoid foods that tear them down.

Drink Right: Drinking uncontaminated water is the only way to stay properly hydrated.

Think Right: Continue to learn, because brain neurons will die if not stimulated.

Move Right: Human bodies were designed to move every day, and people who exercise regularly have healthier bodies and brains.

Sleep Right: Sleep restores our brain and body while poor sleep or not enough sleep increases our risk of dying.

Poop Right: Bowel health determines body health. You need to have at least one easy bowel movement a day.

Talk Right: Optimists have a 42% less risk of death than pessimists. The type of energy that you hold in your body will come out of your mouth.

Firstly, we need to define and understand what it really is to 'detox,' as the term detox has been misused. It has lost its meaning, with many people first thinking of lemon water fasts and juice cleanses being what a detox should be to aid health and weight loss. Also, so much of the time, saying you want to detox could really be you wanting to have a fresh start for your food and lifestyle habits. And if misused, it only fuels the 'quick fix' and obsessive thinking that doesn't get you the long-term results and peace you want.

Dr. David Hawkes put it very well: "Detox" in this context could simply mean eating fresh, healthy food and drinking lots of water. If you put less "junk" into your system, your body has less work to do in breaking it down and getting rid of it."

The benefits that I look for when wanting to aid the body through its natural detox process are:

1. You Feel Better. Quickly getting out of bad habits with food and lifestyle can have you waking up to more energy and clearing away problems such as; brain fog, digestive issues, allergies, and headaches. Your body can become better at producing energy for you to thrive each day.

2. You Lose the Cravings. Many of the problems with cravings are both physiological (your body) and psychological (your brain) working against you. By having an abrupt change in lifestyle and habits around food, it can provide a healthy kickstart to rid the cravings. Then, by also feeding and nourishing your body with the nutrients it needs, it can also help you win the battle of cravings. Though it's not a short-term fix like so many mainstream detox programs, I promise you. And this is why I will show you how this can become an easy everyday thing for you to do.

3. You Lose Weight. By breaking free from the foods that could be causing you to overeat and crave, you can also help balance out insulin and inflammation. Much of the psychological benefit of a well-designed detox program is that when your motivation is highest, it helps you make the changes needed that set you up for long-term success.

So now, let's dive straight into…

How to Detox Your Body.

Firstly, we need to stop the toxins going in. Then we can aid the body to get the toxins out.

Dr. Bob Rokawski and I agreed very much that when it comes to detoxing for health, that it goes beyond just the body. This is also a perfect time to look at what toxins are happening on an emotional and mental level. Immediately, when I was talking with Dr. Bob, I thought of how NOT watching the news has dramatically and positively impacted my life.

Stopping the influx of 'toxins' which could come in the form of bad media, influences, friends, family, and information is going to have a profound effect on you. You being in a better state of mind is only going to lead to better results in your life. How often when you have tried to lose weight, or go after a dream of yours, have naysayers come in with their unwanted opinion;

"Oh, you don't need to do that to lose weight. You just need to…."

This becomes an all too often mantra that is force fed down to you from even well-intentioned loved ones. Everyone wanting to give you their thoughts and advice, when you might not even want it.

So for me, and with our members, we go through 3 steps that help with a 'mental detox.'

#1 - Stop watching the news.

I question the need for knowing the minute-by-minute updates about what's going on around the world. For me, I want to best be able to impact my 'world' that I have a direct influence over, and that's my friends, family, colleagues, and community. When breaking news comes out, I promise you that you will find out about it; It's been shown that major news events have been reported faster via Twitter than on the main news channels.

#2 - Limit Your Social Media.

> "Comparison is the thief of joy"
>
> - Theodore Roosevelt.

This is a brilliant quote that unfortunately wraps up the negative impact of social media in our modern world can have on our brains.

Constantly scrolling through social media, which often leads you to comparing your life with other people's "highlight reels" leaves you feeling a severe lack of something.

My challenge to myself and my members when first starting is only going on social media twice per day. Choose two times, which could be mid-morning and before dinner to do your work on social media. And if you want brownie points, set a timer. This might sound restrictive, but that's a good thing. This is what I want for you. As I promise you will find more time to properly connect with your friends and community by getting more face time with them.

Much of the problem with social media is that it's designed for you to be addicted to it. The notifications can produce a mental high that wants you coming back for more and more. And this also leads to a problem that I saw myself slipping into. And that's not being able to tolerate boredom.

Look at how often it happens that you might be out for coffee or dinner with a friend, they get up to go to the bathroom, and you dash to your phone to see what the updates you've missed. Or, you post a post up, and 10 minutes later, find yourself searching to see who has liked and commented on it. It's the gratification you're looking for with a source that is fleeting. This opens up a problem in that you are constantly looking for stimulus and have a disconnect with yourself.

#3 - Flood Yourself with Greatness.

This is where I want you to focus more. More quality information and influences that help you toward what you want to achieve and the person you want to become.

Choose to read a book, listen to a podcast, or spend time with someone you want to learn from for 30 minutes a day. As hands down, this one point here can be the most beneficial change you can make right now.

This is why I choose to invest so much of my time producing two podcasts, shooting hundreds of videos, and even writing this book. It forces me to be constantly learning and evolving so I can produce value to the world. I am always so much more happier, motivated, and inspired to do more when I flood myself with positive influences.

How to Detox Your Physical Body

Now, we need to stop the toxins from entering your physical body. Your personal environment that includes air pollution, water impurity, and even chemical exposure from your bed, home, deodorants, and the foods you eat all build-up into what's called your 'toxic load.' As a detox is not some heroic event that you have to grind yourself through, it ranges from what happens every day to shortened detoxification events.

Think of a cup as your body's ability to handle toxins. As you fill your cup, your body can naturally detox. Though as you have problems with gut health, your liver, and a lack of proper nutrition, your cup gets smaller. But to compound this effect, if you are constantly being bombarded with toxins, then it's just like adding more water into the cup. Then with a smaller cup, and a stronger flow of toxins, there becomes a point where the water overflows, and this is when you're going to have problems from toxins exposure.

In a study spearheaded by the Environmental Working Group (EWG), researchers at two major laboratories found an average of

200 industrial chemicals and pollutants in umbilical cord blood from babies born in August and September of 2004 in U.S. hospitals. Tests revealed a total of 147 chemicals in the group. Of the 147 chemicals we detected in umbilical cord blood, we know that 180 cause cancer in humans or animals, 217 are toxic to the brain and nervous system, and 208 cause birth defects or abnormal development in animal tests.

I had the huge honor of being able to learn from Dr. Mark Schauss, who is also the author of Achieving Victory Over A Toxic World, which inside he gives a wonderful example of how our toxic load can easily build up.

From waking up in the morning, your toothpaste, water, deodorant, makeup, clothes, food, food containers, the bottle you drink your water out of, your car, and even the air can all contain an array of harmful chemicals that can lead up to a build-up too overwhelming for your body to handle.

The toxic load build-up can include everything from heavy metals like mercury, arsenic, and lead to virtually omnipresent flame retardant compounds called PBDEs to chemicals like phthalates, formaldehyde, PCBs, and bisphenol A (just to name a few). These toxins are invaders, and the body knows it. Some, like the heavy metals, impact neurological functioning, others, like phthalates, disrupt the endocrine balance. PBDEs, at lower levels, can seriously impact thyroid functioning and at higher levels, can impair reproductive and neurological functioning.

While it is impossible to completely eliminate exposure, starting with four simple steps I believe will go a long way toward protecting you:

- Replace your plastic water bottles with glass or stainless steel.
- Keep plenty of plants in the home.
- Wash all your produce, and where possible, buy organic foods.
- Replace dense toxic cosmetics and personal care products with smarter choices. The Environment Working group www.ewg.org is a fantastic resource for this.

Now, it's time for us to help your body go through the natural detox process. And this happens in three phases.

The first phase of detoxification occurs in the liver. The toxin (which is fat soluble) is attached to a vitamin, which still has it as a toxic compound which can cause lots of oxidative damage if not shuttled into phase 2 properly. In Phase 2, the metabolite gets converted to another molecule by the addition of an amino acid or a sulfurous compound. This turns it into a water-soluble compound that's easier to extreme out.

Then in the 3rd Phase, the body is able to extreme the toxin out through urine, faces, or sweat. The problem with so many mainstream 'detox programs' is that phase 1 detox is easy to speed up. The "fruit and vegetable" cleanses can start the Phase 1 process and have you releasing toxins from your fat cells into your bloodstream. But you have a bottleneck problem where you have too much Phase 1, and there is a lack of the amino acids and sulfurous compounds to properly go through Phase 2 detox. This is where you can become even more toxic and cause more problems as the toxins have been released into your bloodstream but are unable to be extorted out of the body.

This is where the importance of your gut health also plays an important role. And why in coming chapters, and the plan, is for you to start focusing on improving your gut health. The GI tract and liver are two primary organs involved with elimination. To help your liver do its job, juice cleanses do one thing right, and that is to provide you with an abundant number of phytonutrients, which come from dark green, blue, purple, and red veggies and fruits. Though why juice cleanses cannot be the ideal solution is because they don't provide you with the amino acids and fiber to help you properly detox.

Four steps to help your liver naturally detox each day, you can:

1: Eat protein rich foods. Your waste product has to be bound with amino acids to be excreted and prevent a build-up of Phase 1 metabolites that can cause more damage.

2: Eat phytonutrient foods: Starting with cruciferous vegetables, these are powerhouses along with the other fruits and veggies that we include in the My Body Diet to nourish you with the antioxidants, phytonutrients, sulfurous compounds, and nutrients that activate detoxification enzymes in the liver.

3: Include natural chelators: These are compounds that bind with heavy metals and other toxins to help extreme them from the body. I personally love including garlic, parsley, and cilantro in my daily meals, which nourish you with natural chelators.

4: Hydrate yourself: It's far too easy to go through a busy day and not drink enough water to properly hydrate yourself. Your body needs to be hydrated to thrive.

This is why I designed the starting 14-Day Metabolic Switch (and the programs after) to be an evidence-based approach to restoring optimal function and health. It's not a crease or a fast. I'm not going to give you lemon juice and maple syrup, or just have you drinking shakes all day long. The goal of the Metabolic Switch is to reduce inflammation, regulate your immune system, super-charge your metabolism, and set you up for long-term success by nourishing you with nutrient-dense foods.

For all new members and private clients, I don't delve into a specific 7-day nutrition cleanse, as it can be overkill in the beginning. This is a tool we use when needed, when the time is right. For you, right now, the most important thing is to use a step-by-step daily practice that will help your body naturally detox and build-up into long-term success.

18

THE 4 SIMPLE STEPS TO LOSING WEIGHT FAST

Here we go, the part of the program where you discover how and why you are going to be able to easily transform your body and health. And how this is going to be done, not by fighting through hunger or cravings or gritting your teeth through endless cardio workouts. No. You're actually going to do it by having confidence in each day and in each action you take. I'm going to show you the 'why' all of this works.

Over the next 14 days and beyond, you're going to go through the first part of your transformation, literally setting you up for success. You're going to be able to do this by tearing down bad habits, but more importantly, replacing them with new empowering habits. You're going to happily go through each day, not second guessing "what or when you should eat," and not having to do the mental math or pull out your calorie tracking app at every meal.

A lot of people, when they go through this, say they feel like they have "regained control." That they no longer are going through each day confused by not knowing what to do and frustrated with not seeing their body change the way they want. But the truth is, you never lost control. No one ever took it from you, you had it all along.

It took me a very long time to finally see this for myself, because as I was trying every diet possible, and especially in the super low-calorie and low-carbohydrate diets, I knew my willpower, focus, and sheer determination would get me through it. Though in truth, it only got me more frustrated, in worse health, and with a slower metabolism. I was blaming all the gurus, authors, and creators of these diets because "they didn't work."

It was when I finally stopped trying to blame everyone else and started to research and find the truth out for myself, that I had the confidence flood over me that the answers have always been here. I just had to go and find them, use them, and perfect them.

This is how I came to what we now use with all members and clients with My Body Blends, and they are the four principles.

1. Eat whole, nutrient-dense foods.
2. Move every day.
3. Bridge your nutrition gap.
4. Upgrade your lifestyle.

And I am going to walk you through each of them right now.

Eat Whole, Nutrient-Dense Foods

Many members now call this eating "fat-loss foods" as this is the side effect that comes from feeding yourself the foods that do four major functions for you.

Firstly, they nourish you with the vitamins, minerals, antioxidants, phytonutrients, fiber, nutrients, and macronutrients you need for your body to thrive. Then they also control your hunger and cravings as they make you full quickly and keep you feeling full for longer.

Thirdly, they provide you with energy but do so that you have an even and balanced day. They then also allow your body to be in a much greater hormonal environment that accelerates your fat loss. With many factors coming together to allow you to burn off the unwanted weight, one of these is because of the controlled blood sugar response.

As you now know, you need two things to have the best fat-loss results. You need a caloric deficit and hormonal balance. Why we have a quality first approach to nutrition rather than a quantity approach (just thinking about counting calories) is because hormones control metabolism. And when insulin, cortisol, leptin, thyroid, and other hormones are 'balanced,' fat loss becomes and an effective and efficient process.

Importantly, it has to be easy for you to follow. This is where we combine the science of what your body needs to burn off the unwanted weight, along with the proven steps and plans to fit this into your lifestyle.

You can now see that when your diet and meal plans have the

above four factors working for you, you're going to be able to break free from the traditional dieting and shape the body and health you want.

Move Every Day

Movement and exercise are two very important factors when it comes to being in the best shape and health you want. Our bodies were made to have lots of movement, and to use the good stress (eustress) of exercise to be able to build stronger, healthier bodies.

Unfortunately, much of the time, there are two sides of the pendulum that most people sit on, and both don't equal the best results. On one side, we have the highly motivated and fitness junkies that can be training too much. The other side has people that either burn out from training so much, or are so confused and even scared of it that they don't do enough training, or none at all.

This is why we use three types of movement and training in our plans to give you the perfect mix that suits what you like, and what gets you to your goals.

Metabolic Resistance Training is the foundation of our workouts, and they can be done 3-5 times a week, as you'll see in the workout plans I give you. This is because it's going to give you the biggest bang for your buck for results.

Then there is Yin Movement. We found the fitness world had completely forgotten about the importance of including this style of movement. We don't really class this as exercise, as you'll see it's really about the calmer yin side compared to the higher intensity yang side. Most fitness gurus are just telling you to smash yourself in every workout, and go harder, harder, harder.

We've found this is not the right balance, and to get great results, it can be a lot easier and more enjoyable. Most people are shocked to find out that just walking is a huge part of my exercise plan. I'll show you how it all works in the coming chapter.

Bridge Your Nutrition Gap

There is no doubt that the common foods we now find in our grocery stores are not providing us with the amount and variety of important nutrients we need.

We have worked hard to now have the simple formula that bridges the gap from what you are getting from your foods; to what will have your body thriving.

From soil depletion to non-organic foods, to farming methods that have sucked the nutrients from our foods, it has now become clear that there are key nutrients that we can easily be lacking. These key nutrients are tied into important metabolic processes that directly tie into your body's ability to burn fat.

Not only are you going to be burning off the unwanted weight easier. You're going to be feeling and performing better as we optimize your body.

Upgrade Your Lifestyle

There are three huge factors that we can make small but powerful changes. Stress, sleep, and mindset.

Firstly, you're going to discover how the habits that we fall into (without consciously knowing) set us up for success or failure. And why, taking you through the key lifestyle factors that set you up for <u>automatic</u> weight loss is a part of the secret sauce why this program works so well.

Then there is your sleep and your stress. Both are tied together, yet individually, can be wreaking havoc on your body. As it's amazing how we can make some changes to what you do 30 minutes before you go to bed, or how dark your bedroom is, or even how 5 minutes of breathing can wash away so many problems.

The science that is coming out now is so strong that it's been a major focus on perfecting the best actions for you to take, and we are proudly going to walk you through it in the upcoming chapter.

Now you know the four important steps and what is behind them, let's dive into how you make it work for you.

19
THE MY BODY DIET

What if you knew exactly how to eat so to shape the body you want?

What if you were able to stop stressing over "am I eating too much?"

And what if you didn't have to follow any stricter rules, calorie numbers, or cut your favorite foods out of your diet?

Well, as you'll soon see, this all starts here, and a simple change of asking a different question changed the entire way I looked at food for fat loss.

So much of the health and fitness world has been focused on quality, which quickly leads into the "more is better" thinking. So, people can easily think well if I should be losing half a pound of fat a week eating this many calories, then I can cut my calories even further to lose more weight.

Or if 45-minute workouts, 4 times a week is what I've been told to do, then 60-minute, or more, workouts every day is what I need to be doing.

This is commonly what's seen in serious physique athletes, and especially, bikini models. And this isn't to give bikini models grief, it's just the truth. I, and other coaches, have had many, bikini models come to us "needing to be fixed," as they've been put through crazy diets and workout plans that have caused metabolic damage.

As the quantity mindset, along with the 'more is better' approach, can have you going down a death spiral of constantly cutting calories and doing more exercise, until you get to the point where you have extreme low-calorie diets, with 1 to 2 hours of exercise a week, and the person just can't lose any weight.

So, let's turn the problem around, and ask a smarter question that has an automatic flow-on effect of positive results.

What if you could improve the quality of your nutrition. Focusing on the foods that have you feeling satisfied, and will nourish your body with the fiber, nutrients, vitamins, minerals, co-factors, and phytochemicals that your body can thrive off and be able to balance important metabolic hormones.

Even the Medical Daily has reported: "Shifting the focus away from calories and emphasizing a dietary pattern that focuses on food quality rather than quantity will help to rapidly reduce obesity, related diseases, and cardiovascular risk." (36)

This is where you're going to get the biggest 'bang for your bite.' As one of the best things that comes with this is the 'automatic' weight loss and health benefits. We've already covered how your hormones play such an important role in your body being able to burn fat off and keep it off.

And this is where by nourishing yourself with the right nutrient-dense foods and having the flexibility also built in your meal plan to still eat your favorite foods, that it's a win/win. And one of the major ways this happens is because you are not obsessing over all the foods you're trying to avoid. Instead, you are just focused on all the foods you can happily eat.

As this used to happen to me all the time, and I always laughed when new clients would confess to the same stories. The typical battle that has you constantly trying to not think about, or willing yourself to not go and get that one food you just want to eat so badly. And just like with the Ben and Jerry's ice cream example I gave in the last chapter, your willpower can cave and easily lead to your binging on the exact foods you were trying to avoid.

By having the foods that work with you on a hormonal and a psychological way, you're not having to go through those battles or binges anymore.

Dr. Joel Fuhrman, author of the book "Eat to Live," coined the now-trendy term "nutritarian," which I think is fantastic. A nutritarian is someone who chooses foods based on their micronutrient per calorie content. This also goes into how you should not follow a "one size fits all" diet plan or theory. Rather, nutritarians focus on eating a variety of unprocessed, whole foods to feel satisfied and remain healthy.

The reason why the My Body Diet is so successful is that it gives you very simple principles to work from. It puts the power back in your own hands to make the changes as you need to. It's also not about getting caught up in all the nitty gritty details that I know you simply don't have the time for.

One of the biggest issues is that most mainstream diets focus on taking foods away, reduction, and depriving you. This is where I want you to focus on eating nutrient-dense foods as, especially, in the first 14-days, it's going to help you bring your appetite and hormones back into balance.

You have an 'automatic' weight loss effect as you naturally start eating less, as you're nourishing yourself with greater nutrients day to day. You have a greater balance with insulin, leptin, and ghrelin so that you're not overeating or cravings the foods that can cause you problems.

Dr. Fuhrman created his own nutrient density formula and scale that are presently patent-pending. He uses 20 different nutrients — including essential vitamins, minerals, **carotenoids**, fiber, and ORAC (antioxidant) scores -- to create a nutrient density standard by which to measure different foods.

This is why, when we choose to eat the majority of our foods from whole, nutrient-dense sources along with the simple PFVC meal model and portion guide, you have a 3-step process to happily put together each meal every day, which have you thriving with health and losing weight that stays off.

20
THE PVFC MEAL MODEL

You do not eat calories.

You do not eat macronutrients.

You eat food.

And this is why we piece together each of your meals with ease using the PVFC meal model.

As when I boil it down to what works so well for my members, who I know are limited with time, want quick results and need a simple plan to follow, these are the basic steps.

And when you understand that, "You can't out run your fork."

We can start with basic changes to your meal plan right now, which will have a big impact on how your body can burn body fat.

Science shows that everything to do with your body burning fat is NOT all about calories in versus calories out. And that your hormones are an important piece of the puzzle.

And one of the most common questions I get when it comes to losing weight is:

"What foods should I be eating?" and…

"How much food should I be eating?"

As we have covered that, yes, you also need to be in a calorie deficit to lose weight. But we know that the "eat less and exercise more" advice, unfortunately, rarely works as the brain has powerful mechanisms for overriding our efforts when we just try to restrict food and exercise more. If you consciously reduce the number of calories you eat, your body responds by lowering your metabolism to match your reduced intake. So, as you purposefully eat fewer calories, your body finds ways to use fewer calories, all while, **ramping up hormones** that raise your appetite and drive you to eat more at every meal so to regain the fat you've lost.

The holy grail for weight loss is an approach that naturally leads to you eating less, without trying to eat less, and happily nourishing your body with the nutrients it needs to thrive each day. This is why I designed the My Body Diet to be satisfying per calorie, which means it's more filling for the same number of calories compared to other popular diet methods. This is crucial for weight loss since it helps you eat less without fighting hunger or counting calories.

Not only do you not have to count calories, you can easily put together each meal and have it fit into your lifestyle. One of the most important factors of any diet or weight loss program is; can you easily stick to it!

This is why we created the PVFC Meal Plan.

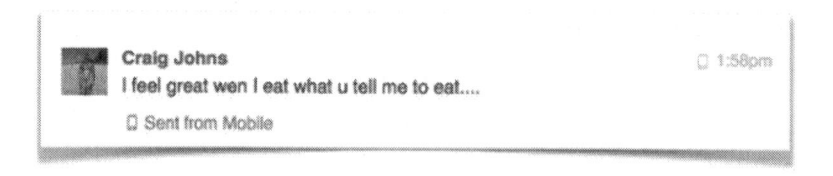

> **Craig Johns** — 1:58pm
> I feel great wen I eat what u tell me to eat....
> Sent from Mobile

This also takes from the "metabolic winter" hypothesis after researching the work of Ray Cronise. (203) This is an exert from The "Metabolic Winter" Hypothesis:

The concept of the "Calorie" originated in the 1800s in an environment with limited food availability, primarily as a means to define economic equivalencies in the energy density of food substrates. Soon thereafter, the energy densities of the major macronutrients--fat, protein, and carbohydrates--were defined.

However, within a few decades of its inception, the "Calorie" became a commercial tool for industries to promote specific food products, regardless of health benefit. Modern technology has altered our living conditions and has changed our relationship with food from one of survival to palatability.

Advances in agriculture, food manufacturing, and processing have ensured that calorie scarcity is less prevalent than calorie excess in the modern world. Yet, many still approach dietary macronutrients in a reductionist manner and assume that isocalorie foodstuffs are isometabolic (203).

Your meals are broken down into:

P = **Protein**

V = **Veggies** (choosing from the All You Can Eat Carb List)

F = **Fats**

C = **Carbs** (your starchy and fruit carbs)

Power Smoothie	Your Power Smoothie can be had for breakfast or to easily replace another meal that includes your macronutrients and micronutrients to fuel the day. **Protein Powder - Superfoods - Fats - Green Veg**
P-V	**Your Protein and Veg meal.** Focussing on just protein and fibrous vegetables and avoiding added fats and carbs in this meal. Use the P-V-F-C Guideline for food choices.
P-V-F	**Your Protein, Veg and Fats meal.** Help boost fat loss and nourish your body with important nutrients including high quality fats. Use the P-V-F-C Guideline for food choices.
P-V-C	**Your Protein, Veg and Carbs meal.** Including starchy carbs to fuel recovery and with the correct timing to help fuel your body and metabolism. Use the P-V-F-C Guideline for food choices.
Refuel Meal	**Refuel your body and brain** with the foods you enjoy with none of the guilt.

We also use smoothies as a quick and easy way to get a strong punch of nutrition that tastes great and can be easily put together when on the run.

Hundreds use this as a great breakfast option or a meal during the busy day. You can use our Low Carb Breakfast Smoothie or our Green Smoothie recipes that are found in the free Bonus Downloads - http://mybodyblends.com/freebook.

To know what foods you can eat, I've also included a shopping list for you (download it in the free guides section):

SHOPPING LIST. The My Body Diet.

MEAT/PROTEIN
- ☐ Chicken Breast
- ☐ Turkey
- ☐ Beef Steak
- ☐ Lean Pork Chops
- ☐ Eggs
- ☐ Chicken Thigh
- ☐ Kangaroo
- ☐ Lamb
- ☐ Pork Mince
- ☐ Chicken Mince
- ☐ Beef Mince
- ☐ Veal Mince
- ☐ Turkey Mince
- ☐ Salmon
- ☐ Crab
- ☐ Prawns
- ☐ Snapper
- ☐ John Dory
- ☐ Blue Eye Cod
- ☐ Lobster
- ☐ Scallops
- ☐ Anchovy
- ☐ Sea Bass
- ☐ Halibut

FRUITS
- ☐ Lime
- ☐ Lemon
- ☐ Blueberries
- ☐ Strawberries
- ☐ Blackberries
- ☐ Kiwi Fruits
- ☐ Oranges
- ☐ Pear
- ☐ Apple
- ☐ Peach
- ☐ Papaya
- ☐ Watermelon

FIBROUS VEGETABLES
- ☐ Tomato
- ☐ Avocado
- ☐ Spinach
- ☐ Baby Spinach
- ☐ Cabbage
- ☐ Broccoli
- ☐ Celery
- ☐ Watercress
- ☐ Asparagus
- ☐ Zucchini
- ☐ Cucumber
- ☐ Red Onion
- ☐ Carrots
- ☐ Kale
- ☐ Snow Peas
- ☐ Capsicum
- ☐ Beets
- ☐ Cauliflower
- ☐ Bok Choy
- ☐ Garlic

STARCHY CARBS
- ☐ Sweet Potato
- ☐ Yam
- ☐ Pumpkin
- ☐ Brown Rice
- ☐ Quinoa
- ☐ Beans
- ☐ Lentils

DRINKS
- ☐ Green Tea
- ☐ Herbal Tea
- ☐ Water

FROZEN FOODS
- ☐ Blueberries
- ☐ Mixed Berries
- ☐ Mixed Vegetables

FATS
- ☐ Olive Oil
- ☐ Flaxseed Oil
- ☐ Macadamia Oil
- ☐ Coconut Oil
- ☐ Fish Oil
- ☐ MCT Oil
- ☐ Almonds
- ☐ Walnuts
- ☐ Brazil Nuts
- ☐ Macadamia
- ☐ Pecans
- ☐ Sunflower Seeds
- ☐ Pepitas
- ☐ Cashews

FLAVOUR
- ☐ Basil
- ☐ Ginger Powder
- ☐ Cumin
- ☐ Chili Powder
- ☐ Turmeric
- ☐ Oregano
- ☐ Parsley
- ☐ Cocoa Powder
- ☐ Lime Juice
- ☐ Organic
- ☐ Salsa
- ☐ Stevia
- ☐ Mint
- ☐ Dill
- ☐ Cinnamon
- ☐ Paprika
- ☐ Cayenne Pepper
- ☐ Black Pepper
- ☐ Sea Salt
- ☐ Minced Garlic
- ☐ Ginger
- ☐ Chili Flakes

MISCELLANEOUS
- ☐ Butter
- ☐ Vanilla Extract
- ☐ Apple Cider Vinegar
- ☐ Balsamic Vinegar
- ☐ Rosemary
- ☐ Pinto Beans
- ☐ Honey
- ☐ Vinegar
- ☐ Pea Protein Powder
- ☐ Steel Cut Oats

Here is an easy to use list of foods so you can put your meals together.

Protein	Veggies	Fats	Carbs
Chicken Breast	Cabbage	Coconut Oil	Sweet Potato
Turkey Breast	Broccoli	Olive Oil	Brown Rice
Beef	Spinach	Macadamia Nut Oil	Oats
Venison	Celery	Avocado	Quinoa
Lamb	Watercress	Nuts and Seeds	Beans
Kangaroo	Asparagus	Butter	Lentils
Salmon	Tomato		
White Fish	Zucchini		
Prawns	Cucumber		
Pork	Onion		
Whole Eggs	Snow Peas		
	Bok Choy		

The Quality of Your Food

<u>"You are not what you eat. You're are what you eat, ate."</u>

Now, if I don't talk about the quality of your foods and meats, then I wouldn't be able to sleep at night. Let's use the example of grass-fed versus grain-fed meat. Organic, grass-fed meat provides more nutrients and fewer toxins than grain-fed or conventional meat. Organic, grass-fed meat also has more antioxidants, Omega 3's, trace minerals, vitamins and conjugated linoleum acid (CLA), which is a type of naturally occurring fat that improves brain function, causes weight loss and can reduce your risk of cancer.

In the case of meat, you see that the animal eats vegetables, which it then uses the amino acids to build protein. This means that we can then eat the animal to get a greater, and dense source of the protein.

> **Jenny** — 6 August 2014 8:29 pm
> This is 3rd morning of my program and already seeing results...bloat gone and already leaning out in abs... Seeing results helps the motivation and food cravings... Lol Thanks Chris:)

> **Lindsay Brewer** ▶ Fit Body Pro I Members Online
> 10 hrs · Caloundra
> Week 1 almost up on the Total Transformation Program and what can I say but WOW! Feel more lively, much stronger and looked leaner when I woke up this morning. Can't wait to take measurement and photos.

Protein

Each time we sit down to a meal, we put our protein on the plate first. And for good reason.

One example is this study, which showed that the high-protein group lost significantly more fat mass compared to the low protein group, even though both groups ate the same number of calories. (202) I see this being due to greater meal satisfaction and less hunger. Planning meals around high-quality proteins is a method that is well researched for fat loss.

The mainstream media has you confused with the pendulum of advice swinging from one radical side to the other. We have the ketogenic crowd saying that a lower protein intake of 10-20% of total energy consumption is good. At the same time, we have anti-aging sources stating that a protein restriction and fasting approach can lower mTOR. MTOR is an ancient molecular signaling pathway that is responsible for either growth or repair, depending on whether it is stimulated or inhibited. This is obviously a needed mechanism in the body, but science is starting to show that over stimulus with a high-protein, and high food intake can cause problems with aging.

But again, I see that the truth lays somewhat in the middle and that it's dependent on yourself and your goals. This is also another reason, why I generally recommend a broader eating window, where an Intermittent Fasting approach is used, so that you cycle mTOR activation, both being able to benefit from its effects when high and low.

At the time of writing, I am also experimenting with having one day a week where I do not eat any animal products. As I see it, our bodies have evened from the standpoint of not always constantly consuming foods, and types of foods each and every day. Personally, at this point, I'm really enjoying it and find it helpful with digestion and being able to stay lean with high energy. However, I've personally not done enough work into this to add it into the program. Thus, why I recommend you join the free group and get the Bonus Downloads, so you get all the updates that are to come:

cravingthetruth.com/bookbonus

Vegetables

The My Body Diet is high in nutrient-rich vegetables. As one thing that the very, very large majority of experts in the health and wellness space ranging from vegetarians to meat lovers say, is that we should all eat more vegetables.

This is the food 'type' that you're going to be eating the most of. And note that I separate vegetables from starchy carbs and fruits.

I don't just put all of them under the one umbrella of foods like so many other diet programs do.

This is because they are very different! The My Body Diet focuses on vegetables with the highest nutrient density and lower antinutrient load. This nourishes you with your micronutrient needs that don't come from your animal products. Plus, as you now know, the importance of fiber and how first focusing on protein and vegetables is going to keep you fuller for longer, leaving little need or want to consume foods that are loaded with sugar and refined carbohydrates.

Fats

It was when I first interviewed Ryan Munsey for The Limitless Body Podcast that breaking news came out via the New York Times. The sugar industry had paid off scientists in the 1960's to downplay the health problems associated with sugar and put the cause onto saturated fat (204). "They were able to derail the discussion about sugar for decades," said Stanton Glantz, a professor of medicine at U.C.S.F. and an author of the JAMA Internal Medicine paper.

And just like with all foods, there are differences in quality, and there are some "bad" fats that really will make you sick and fat. But when you include the right amounts of the right types of fat, such as what I have for you in the meal plan, you will be nourishing yourself with key nutrients.

Our cells, organs, and brains are all made of fat and need high-quality fat to function optimally.

Along with the sources of fats, I want to give you some simple guidance, which has proved to be very effective for myself and so many members.

The fats that I love to include are; animal fats such as bone marrow, and grass-fed cows, along with coconut oil, whole, eggs, ghee, butter, olive oil, fish oils, and cacao butter.

When it comes to nuts, I'd always rather replace nuts with choices of fats that are from the above list as, let's be perfectly honest, even when we're not counting calories, or looking at portion control, a bag of macadamias or cashews can disappear in a few handfuls without you even noticing, which can lead to these being a trigger food, but also a food that could be replaced with another choice that gives you great satiety and enjoyment.

Also with oils, such as olive, macadamia, almond, and walnuts oils is that they can easily become oxidized and be harmful due to heat, light, and air exposure. The foods need to be high-quality and packaged properly, otherwise, you could be buying a rancid product that is only ailing you.

Carbs

The simplicity in which Shelby Starnes can explain the complex matters and methods that he uses to so successfully to transform the physiques of his clients is nothing short of brilliant.

And it was why I have interviewed Shelby on numerous occasions to peel back and explain many strategies that can be used for beginner weight loss plans to advanced physique models and bodybuilders preparing to step onto the stage.

One such topic that we have frequently talked about is 'carb cycling.' Shelby describes carb cycling: "By fluctuating macronutrients on a daily basis, we can ensure that performance and muscle building can be optimized on the days when it's most important, while burning fat on the other days."

Carb cycling, when done correctly, gives you the best of both worlds and worst of neither. You are able to fuel your body from your workouts and stimulate your metabolism, but heighten your body's process to be more effective at burning body fat by crashing your metabolism.

This is why we use the PFVC meal model, because it allows you to easily know when to time your nutrients to further acerbate your fat loss without the confusion or hassle that so many advanced fat-loss programs have you scratching your head over.

The My Body Diet is not a low-carb diet. It's not a high-carb diet. It's a smart carb approach, to suit YOU. You'll see that the starting 14-Day Metabolic Switch phase does not have carbs coming from starches or fruit. This is to help reset your metabolism, as I will show you how to do in part 3 of this book. As by getting so many micronutrients and nourishing yourself with the high-quality proteins, vegetables, and fats, you lower your need for consuming starches, such as sweet potato, yams, pumpkins, and legumes.

Then as we teach your body to use carbs effectively, to fuel your life without the spillover effect of fat gain, you will be able to eat more and lose more weight.

We find there is generally a rule of thumb that the more carbs you can tolerate, the less fats you need. So we start with a higher fat, lower carb approach. And often, the carb intake increases and fat intake slightly decreases as your body progresses. Yet there are many factors that influence your body's ability to handle carbohydrates. Two main factors are your training and stress.

If you're weight training more often, and with higher amounts of work done in each session, then your body can generally tolerate, and may need more, carboy dates. Also, if you're experiencing higher amounts of stress, I generally see a decrease in the body's ability to tolerate carbs, and therefore, they are replaced by a higher fat intake.

Rather than making it a complex task of trying to understand everything, and not even knowing how your body is going to handle the changes to come, I would much rather give you the best starting guide now. And then, as you progress along, have the coaching guides show you how to easily change and adapt your diet and training to suit your progress and lifestyle.

This is why I highly recommend you join the free group and get access to the free bonus guides at

cravingthetruth.com/bookbonus

The Low Down on Fruit

Fruit has been kicked around because of its link with fructose. Fructose is a sugar that is metabolized differently in the body, and fructose causes problems because of the immense use of it in foods such as sodas, baked goods, doughnuts, and many processed foods. However, fruit in its whole form provides, water, fiber, and nutrition along with the small amount of fructose that comes with a whole piece of fruit.

My general recommendation is one piece of one serving of fruit a day, and to generally stick with the fruits that I've included in the foods list for you. These fruits are the most nutritious and lowest in anti-nutrients and fructose.

Now when answering "what foods do I eat?" the concept of 'fat-loss foods' gets thrown around online all too often to bait you into clicking on a video or article.

"The Death of Fat Burning Foods"

No… We're not going to talk about magical foods that are "minus calories" or that strip fat off your body as soon as you start munching on them. Instead, we are going to focus on foods that are going to control your hunger and nourish your body with the nutrients it needs to thrive. As when you eat a normal meal, you are shutting down your 'fat burning.' Especially when eating carbs and protein, you will have an insulin response, but also, because you're feeding your body energy that it can burn rather than its own body fat.

However, I'm not going to talk about eating "healthy foods," as that term really means something different to each person. And we now know that: **To lose fat, it takes two things; an energy deficit, and secondly with it being in the context of hormonal balance. The hormonal balance has to come first, and when it does, calorie intake normally takes care of itself.**

So if you eat more of the right things, more often, you're not going to be hungry, not have cravings, and enjoy long stretches of predictable energy. This can automatically control the amount of food you eat. However, the flip side, if you take a calorie first approach, can likely increase hunger and have you wanting to eat more of the foods that continue the fat storing spiral. This can also lower your body's ability to burn body fat as you can be burning calories and losing weight, but if the hormonal balance is off, those calories and that weight will just as likely be coming from muscle as opposed to fat.

These are going to be foods that are rich in protein, fiber, water, and nutrient dense. These help to balance out your energy and blood sugar levels so that you can go for longer stretches of time without getting hungry or needing a boost in energy. This is why the My Body Diet starts with two distinct phases; to fast-track you in finding out what works for you.

21
ANSWERING: HOW MUCH DO I EAT?

The truth is… Counting calories sucks.

When you're trying to count calories, it's a myriad of websites, apps, and math that can make your head spin each day just trying to keep up. And the worst thing, other than how complicated it is, is that research shows those calorie numbers can be wrong by 25%.

All that hard work and math can be totally wrong in the first place. Then you have the other side of the calories in vs. calories out equation. Trying to calculate your 'burned calories' from your exercise and basal metabolic rate, which again, can be wrong by up to 25%.

The "too hard" factor makes it impossible for this to fit into your lifestyle and it's why so many people give up, and the constant yo-yo dieting continues.

The Good News:

There is a much easier way for you to go through each day, nourishing yourself and being able to watch your body change the way you want it to.

Because this book is more about demystifying dieting and the "how to" for weight loss once and for all. This is about how you can get lean and healthy… for the rest of your life.

Even better, you're going to enjoy it.

But before we go into how you can overcome one of the biggest lifestyle issues that can easily be won: "how much do I eat?" let's be very clear on one important fact.

We covered in the earlier chapter "Calories matter… I just don't count them" the importance of energy balance. Simply put, the relationship between the amount of energy you consume and the amount you burn.

The 'hormone only' approach with the forced focus of eating fewer carbs controls insulin, which therefore, limits your fat gain potential isn't the entire picture. It's not an either-or scenario. We need to use both. And we can easily use both.

But after working with clients all around the world, there is a common problem when it comes to controlling and understanding how much food you should eat.

When you're a kid, being a member of the clean plate club is practically a parent's dream come true. "Finish all your dinner, because there are starving kids" or some sort of persuasion tactic is commonly used. But when you're an adult with a bad case of portion distortion, your habit of eating everything in front of you is likely making it impossible for you to lose weight.

This really struck me with my first daughter, Arlo. I've found that she's had this innate ease of being able to just eat what best suits her. And that being that the amount of food, and the foods she is drawn to can differ. Both my wife, Lauren, and I have been conscious to not badger her to eat more from the very beginning. As we were both brought up with the "finish all your food" mentality.

And then it really became clear. "Where did we all go wrong with not being able to know how much to eat, and now overeating is such an epidemic."

Multiple studies spanning decades have proven the link between large portions, overeating, and obesity (197).

Basically, the larger the portions of food you're generally served or serve yourself, the more likely you are to eat too much and gain weight. Thanks to what researchers refer to as a "mindless margin," it's very easy to slightly under- or overeat without realizing it (198).

From plates becoming bigger, and when you go and eat out "normal" portion sizes getting oversized. I also believe the constant battering of our body and minds with the engineered foods that are causing us to now struggle. And this is why, when you start to use a simple method like the PVFC meal model, along with this portion control guide, that your life can become so much simpler.

And more often than not, it becomes a simple habit that you stop having to think about. You don't have to go throughout your entire life with a calorie counting app in your hand or doing the mental math at each meal. You're going to be able to happily eat the foods that best fit you, and eat the amount of the food that best nourishes you.

It amazes me each how much I learn from my own children. And especially, becoming a father and having the opportunity to give my children the best possible start to life, had me want to equip myself with all the information and tools to make this happen.

And a perfect example of what happened just last night, like so many other nights.

Being able to shop, prepare, cook, and have ready dinner to bring the family together each night isn't an easy task, especially with small children, Lauren and I laugh at how it becomes a dance to have everything come together in time to be sure that the bath, story, and bedtime routine happens to make sure the girls are nourished, happy, and off for a great night's sleep.

So yesterday we went to the local farmers market to get some extra food, especially for dinner. The joy of being able to cook with the family around is something I've always enjoyed, as it is a great time to teach our children not only where food comes from, but to have an environment where we can spend time together and talk. But after getting it all together, it's time to serve.

First, we put all the food out on the platters in the middle of the table. I don't want to serve an amount of food in front of them that I think is right for them. I let them, and their hunger and intuition, determine how much they put on their plate and eat. Watching how intuitive children are with their food amazes me. It's the body working as it should, and especially when it's not bombarded with the bad foods that cause cravings and hunger.

Secondly, Arlo, our eldest daughter, sits down and happily says "I'm not hungry." Now to be honest, my first reaction is to say, "eat your dinner darling." That would be the influence of my own growing up and have parents wanting me to be a part of the "clean plate club," ensuring I eat all my dinner. But that, to me, isn't the right reaction. I take a deep breath, get back into the moment, and say, that it's all "ok." As long as she can sit with us and be involved with the conversation, I'm happy. She can choose to eat when she feels like it.

Now, if you're thinking that sounds great but come on Chris, that's not realistic, then I understand why you're saying that. And this is why the My Body Diet is designed the way it is. It's to give you the starting plan that kick-starts your results, and have you break free from the hunger and cravings that have plagued you so far. But more importantly, the plan has you making smarter choices.

There is no - Off or On with the diet. If you decide to eat the foods that could cause you brain fog, cause you to crave sugars or more foods, increase inflammation, or just have you not performing the way you want, that's your choice. You haven't fallen off, and you don't need to start back on the diet. You just make the best choice next, and move on with your life.

To make this really practical so you can make the easy shift from today, let's walk you through how to put your next meal together.

For example, when you have a P-V-F meal, you know your meal is quickly broken into a protein, vegetables, and a fat. It's easy to choose the right foods to fit, so this can be chicken with a mixed salad and nuts with seeds.

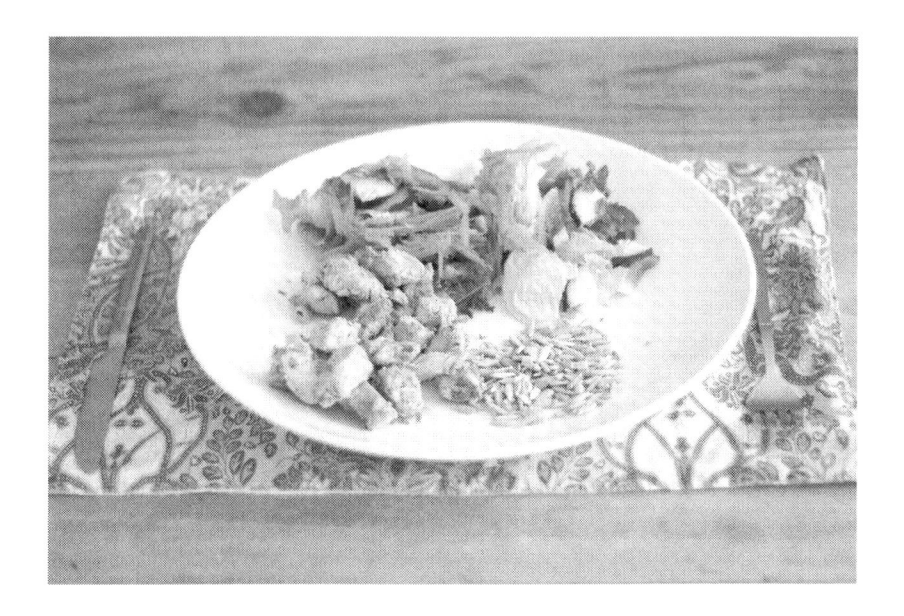

Here is an example meal of Chicken and Salad with Nuts and Seeds

Obviously, your combination of food choices is endless, as the food choice guidelines we give you make sure you have the variety to eat the foods you enjoy.

Though the question of "how much food do I eat?" will come up next. And this is where I thank John Beradi and Precision Nutrition for their simple model.

Here is how it works:

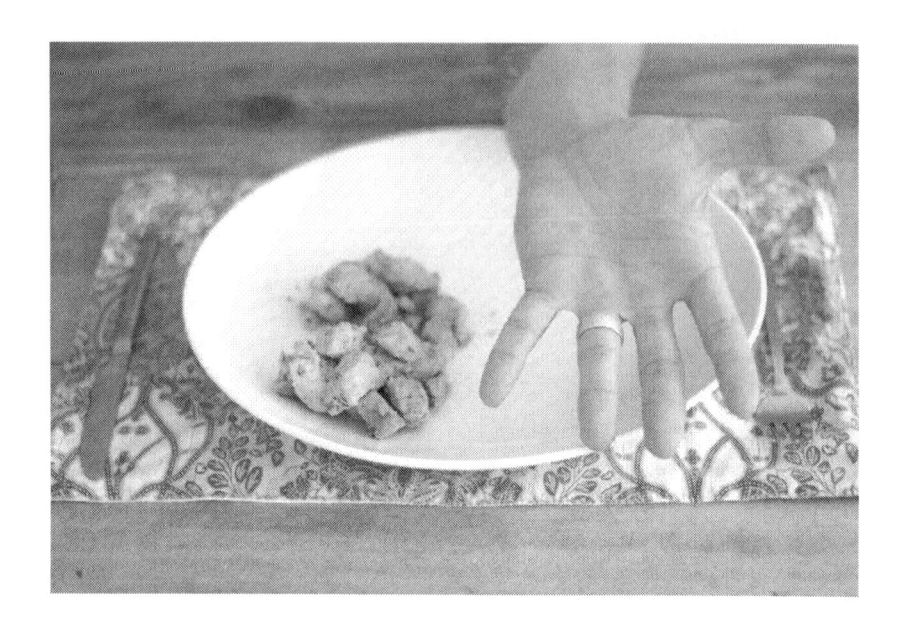

Your palm determines your protein.

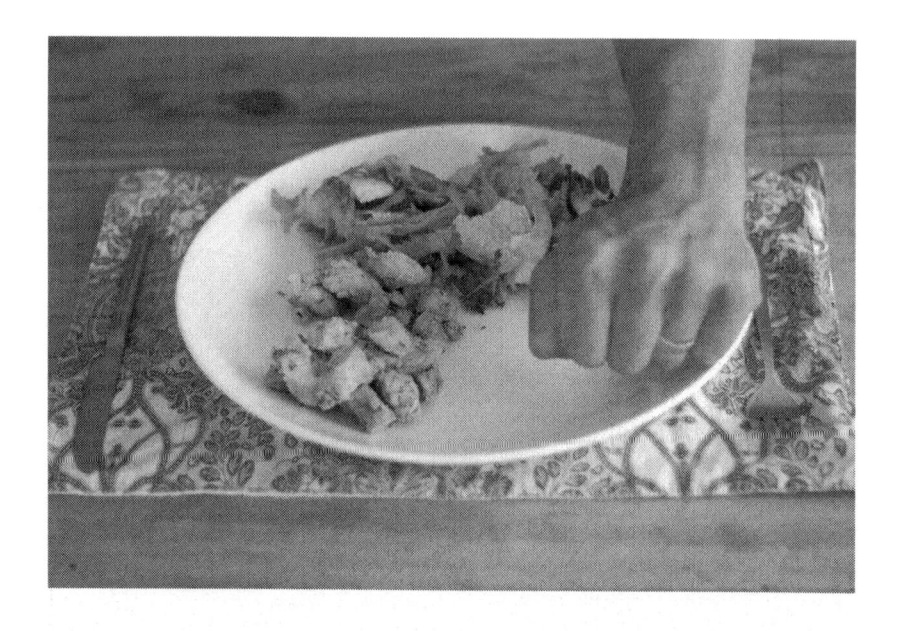

Your fist determines your veggies.

Answering: How Much Do I Eat? 179

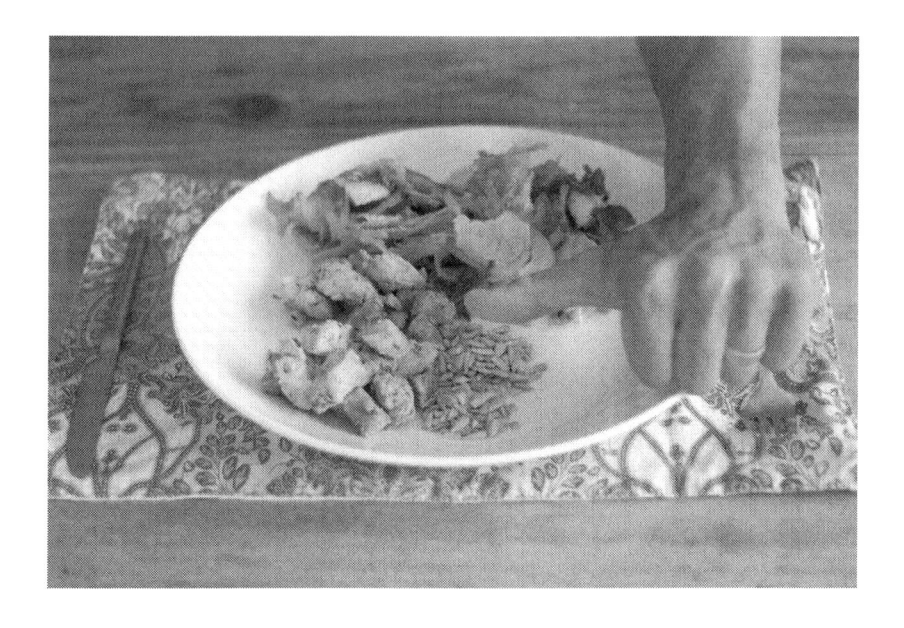

Your thumb determines your fat.

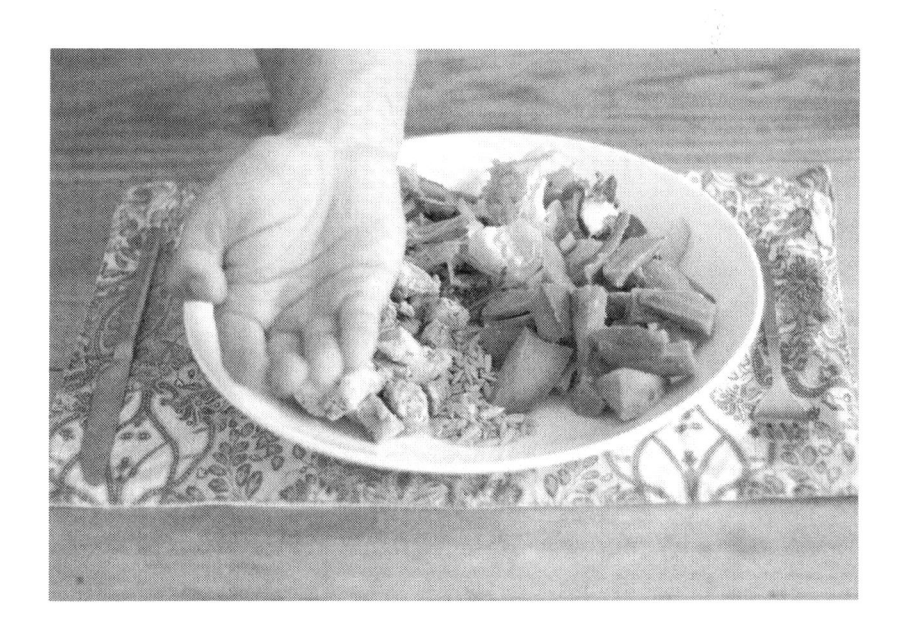

Your cupped hand determines your carbs.

For the starting difference between Men and Women, I've boiled it down to:

For Men:
2 palms of protein with each meal.
2 fists of vegetables with each meal.
2 cupped hands of carbs for selected meals.
2 entire thumbs of fat with selected meals.

For Women:
1 palm of protein with each meal.
1 fist of vegetables with each meal.
1 cupped hand of carbs for selected meals.
1 entire thumb of fat with selected meals.

Now many clients that have been through the calorie and macronutrient counting plans usually say at this point, "Chris, is this accurate enough?" And the simple answer is yes! This isn't a "to the very gram" method. But that's also the reason that we use it. We don't need to be to the very gram and granular with the amounts.

We can then also use the changes in your meal plan to adjust the number of macronutrients you eat, or even the timing of those macronutrients as needed, in a simple way.

When you know what your meals are made of using the PVFC, you can easily 'portion size' your foods, meal prep and quickly put together your meals and know it matches what's needed to give you the body want.

And this is where your new journey starts, and why I give you the starting two-week meal plan. But it's only the starting two weeks. It's not forever, because you're going to easily be able to make changes for your individual needs.

Too hungry? Too full? Not satisfied? Or even if you start training less or more, you can start to adapt your meals and how you eat around how your body is responding and around your life.

22
CHOOSE YOUR EATING WINDOW

We now know that you do not need to eat small, frequent meals throughout the day to "stoke" your metabolism.

This is one reason why we use Intermittent Fasting (IF). And if you're worried because I just said the 'f' word – fasting, it's ok, because my first response when someone tried to tell me to start fasting so that I can burn fat, build muscle, and dramatically improve my health. My answer was:

Are You Serious…?

…but, my metabolism will drop, and I'll lose muscle if I'm not eating!"

This was soon to become the end of the dogmatic, closed mind that was holding me back, not only as a coach, but also in numerous areas of my life.

Now, I've been using fasting in many forms and experimenting with different protocols, and I can see the tremendous benefits that are not only for fat-loss results, but brain cognition and clarity of thinking throughout the days and health benefits, especially with gut health.

Personally, I used an Intermittent Fasting protocol to get to the leanest I've ever been. Prepping for my last fitness model competition, I was far leaner and had retained much more muscle mass months out from the competition. And best of all, it was the easiest approach I had done.

Now, myself and all the members that use this approach are able to stay lean all year round, and not be caught up with the constant stress and thinking of food. One of the greatest benefits is the liberation of food. You realize that once your nourishing and feeding your body with the foods it thrives on when following the My Body Diet, you're not going to be hungry or craving foods throughout the day.

More importantly, the way we answer, "how many meals should I be eating?" is by having an <u>eating window.</u>

My focus for you, and for me, is being able to stay in shape and live with optimal health and energy to be the best version we can be.

If you're like me, you're busy. You want to live a social life, and you don't want to be all consumed constantly thinking of when your next meal is going to come, and what you're going to be eating.

Personally, I run two businesses, I have two beautiful daughters and a wife that I want to be spending lots of quality time with and would like to enjoy life to the fullest.

On a day to day basis, I use some 'form' of Intermittent Fasting, and in this guide, I'm going to walk you through the different types of Intermittent Fasting and how you can start to use it effectively.

The truth is, the term "Intermittent Fasting" is very ambiguous. Just not eating while you sleep could be a 'form' of fasting. Though we are going to look at the physique and health benefits that are beyond this.

We use the term eating window simply to have an easy understanding of when you're eating and when you're not.

Personally, I wake up around 5:30am each day. I like to be able to do my creative work very early, have a short walk, spend time with my family, and have the vast majority of the tasks in hand to running my businesses by midday.

Somewhere between 11am and 2pm, for the past 6 months, I've been having my first meal. The main benefit that I have from this is that I don't have one thought about food for the entire morning.

Plus, there are now proven benefits for being able to go through a fasted period for both body and brain.

Throughout talking with many experts such as Ryan Munsey who has easily been able to make the simple changes to his diet to have a lifestyle that gives him greater performance in the gym and life, physique changes, and brain power.

Plus, having years of experimenting with myself and with clients, I've been able to get great results by using a metabolic flexibility method for program and diet design to enhance fat-loss results.

As there are a 'metabolic' phase and an 'anabolic' phase to each day. This is where we can focus on accelerating fat loss in the metabolic phase, and this is where Intermittent Fasting can be very useful, then in the anabolic phase, using the power of insulin and other hormones to repair, recovery and build lean muscle.

Intermittent fasting is NOT a diet. It's a simple structure to fit the best meal plan that works for you in.

Fasting has no standard duration or strict plan on "how to do it." This is where I want to walk you through this guide, so that you can use fasting from a range of protocols to best suit you.

As it's just a way of scheduling your meals, so it's changing 'when' you eat, not 'what' you eat. This lifestyle change has multiple beneficial effects, which really just come about from very small behavioral changes.

So let's look at why you might want to start this…

There are two main benefits of using an Intermittent Fasting plan:

1 – It gives you a smaller time window in which to eat, which can naturally curb your calorie and energy intake. All "diets" essentially control one or more factors that are to do with limiting calorie intake and/or managing key metabolic hormones to accelerate fat loss and limit fat gain.

We can break this down further into:

– Blood levels of insulin significantly drop, which help facilitate fat burning.

– Increase in Human Growth Hormone, which again, helps facilitate fat burning and other benefits.

2 – There are multiple 'health' benefits, such as having a longer window of time to aid in the proper digestion of food. The increase of autophagy which is the physiological process that your body goes through to have cellular clean up.

And there are also beneficial changes in several genes and molecules related to longevity and protection against disease.

There are two other important benefits, which for me, are a HUGE positive.

1) It makes your day much simpler.

You will set your eating window to begin with at 10 hours. For if you have your first meal at 10am, then your last meal will be at 8pm.

If you feel more comfortable or if it fits your life schedule to eat morning in the morning and finish earlier, then an example would be to have your first meal at 7am and finish at 5pm.

Simply, you have the power to choose what best fits with you and for you to have the guiding principles to make it as easy and as effective.

Also, as you'll see in the chapter of 'The Death of Cheating,' I believe in the power of the words we use. Breakfast, is simply to 'break' the 'fast.' This also empowers you to eat what you want at each meal.

2) Brain power and clarity can be much higher due to a fasted state. To back this up and give you the real-world insights I interviewed Tyler Tolman and Jimmy Moore who were both featured on the Limitless Body Podcast.

Two very different perspectives on why they were using a larger eating window that mimics an Intermittent Fasting approach. And both getting fantastic results. Yet both were very concise with not only the benefits of it for the body, but also the function and performance of the brain.

This is also why I love this quote from Dr. Michael Eades –

> Diets are easy in the contemplation, difficult in the execution. Intermittent fasting is just the opposite -- it's difficult in the contemplation but easy in the execution. Most of us have contemplated going on a diet. When we find a diet that appeals to us, it seems as if it will be a breeze to do. But when we get into the nitty gritty of it, it becomes tough. For example, I stay on a low-carb diet almost all the time. But if I think about going on a low-fat diet, it looks easy. I think about bagels, whole wheat bread and jelly, mashed potatoes, corn, bananas by the dozen, etc. -- all of which sound appealing. But were I to embark on such a low-fat diet I would soon tire of it and wish I could have meat and eggs. So a diet is easy in contemplation, but not so easy in the long-term execution.
>
> Intermittent fasting is hard in the contemplation, of that there is no doubt. "You go without food for 24 hours?" people would ask, incredulously when we explained what we were doing. "I could never do that." But once started, it's a snap. No worries about what and where to eat for one or two out of the three meals per day. It's a great liberation. Your food expenditures plummet. And you're not particularly hungry. … Although it's tough to overcome the idea of going without food, once you begin the regimen, nothing could be easier.

-- Dr. Michael Eades

Before we dive into how easily you can be setting up your own meal plan and eating window that suits you, let me give you two examples of what I use at the moment…

The Two Types of Fasting I Use Each Week (and you can too)

16-8

The popular 16 hours fasting, and an 8-hour window of eating was brought to my attention through Martin Berkhan of Leangains.

I usually eat my last meal around 7 to 8pm, which means the 16-hour fasting window ends at 11am-2pm the next day. This does look like a glorified way of skipping breakfast.

BUT… it gives you the great benefits that I mentioned above.

At this point, I've been doing it long enough that I just go by how I feel. You'll also see below the how and why in which you can easily use this type of method.

Though I also understand as a coach, I need to equip you with the tools and power to take the best and smartest action for yourself. This is why, in the meal plans I give you with this book, that there can be a set structure and help for you to progress as you go.

The truth is, you're going to have to try this yourself to see if it works for you. I'll also outline the key points for to you to follow in the 'secret sauce' section below for you to start this properly.

Let me give you an example that Lauren, my wife, is using at the moment.

She likes to train in the morning after one of us drops our eldest daughter off at school, which means her training session starts around 8:30 to 9am.

Her training plan usually involves 3-4 weight training sessions per week, with 1-2 intervals of bodyweight sessions included as well.

So, she will start with a black coffee before she leaves the house, and has her water bottle with BCAA (branch chain amino acids) to start sipping throughout her workout. This means that by the time she gets home, showers, and has fed our youngest daughter it's about 10:30am before she can sit down and have her first meal.

This is where Lauren first started experimenting with the Bulletproof Coffee that was created from Dave Asprey. When we first started having a larger window from last meal to first meal, we found that including a Bulletproof Coffee before her workouts gave her the brain power and satiety to easily extend her fast for longer.

As we have dinner at around 7pm, this is a fasting window of 15 and a half hours from meal to meal.

In times where I follow more of an "eat less, move less" scenario (that was taught to me from Jade Teta), I've been using a Bulletproof Coffee around midday to easily have my first meal between 1-3pm. The quality fats, especially the use of proper MCT oil, can help fuel brain function and keep off hunger.

Personally, my favorite variation of the Bulletproof Coffee is 1 teaspoon of butter, 1 teaspoon of MCT oil, and a pinch of cinnamon blended together with high-grade coffee.

The 24 Hour Fast

As I delved deeper into the research and talked with numerous experts from around the world as I brought them onto the My Body Blends Podcast, the longer extended fasts we're looking to give some great benefits.

Especially after living and working in Dubai, I coached many local Emirates including Arab Sheiks that were going through Ramadan. Leading into the first Ramadan I experienced there, I poured into the research to learn how best to train and coach my clients going through an extended fast. This is where my interest in fasting first came about.

The 24-hour fast I do once a week is simple:

Let's say I eat dinner on Saturday night at 7pm.

I won't eat again until 7pm on Sunday night (told you it was simple).

I enjoy doing the extended fast once a week, as on those Sundays I am 100% focused on family time.

On this day, I don't do any weight or intense training. My movement for the day would be my daily morning walk, and if I can get a surf or a short yoga or stretching session in, I'm winning!

It's all about progress…

No way am I going to expect you to jump straight into a 24-hour, or even a 16-hour, fast from tomorrow.

Personally, the actual time isn't the main predictor of how long I am going too fast for.

It was by learning from Tyler Tolman the 3 different 8-hour cycles that the body will go through in a 24-hour period (detoxification from 4am-12 noon, appropriation 12noon-8pm and assimilation 8pm-4am), was what had me decide on experimenting, which has now turned into a daily habit of eating at the times I do. However, I also just see these as guidelines to empower you to make smarter choices that best serve you.

This is important: and how you can free yourself from 'diets.'

The Anti-Douche Guide to Intermittent Fasting

Where I see Intermittent Fasting become a stress and a strain in life is when people try to use willpower, and push past when they shouldn't. All you need to understand is that some days you will do better, and some days you won't.

The simple changes that go on with your body and environment determine what your body needs with its foods and how you can tolerate stress.

Let's say I choose to do a 16-hour fast tomorrow, but tonight, my youngest daughter (who is 7 months old at the moment) has woken up a few times during the night.

The lack of quality and quantity of sleep means my stress tolerance and blood sugar management the next day is impaired. So there's a good chance that I'm just not going to be able to handle an extended fast, which means I'll happily eat throughout the day.

If I start to become "hangry" (the combination of angry and hungry) and am becoming a douche bag of a father, husband, or dude – then the fast ends, I eat, and get on with life.

There is zero need to get bummed out about it…

There is also the question that comes up with fasting and how it affects your metabolic rate. Especially, people worrying about if it's going to lower their metabolic rate, and hurt their ability to lose weight and keep it off.

It's been shown that after 36 hours of fasting, an increase in metabolic rate is seen, which does not change further when measured at 72 hours (47). Also shown is that in non-obese people, alternate day fasting (where you are eating every other day) does not result in a decrease in metabolic rate after 22 days. And this is when they were instructed to eat twice as much food on the days they could eat. So overall, there was no calorie drop (48).

Firstly, I don't use alternate day fasting as I've found it really uncomfortable, and so did the clients I tested it with. I found no need to continue using it. Though the above science does show that we can use intentional fasting for many benefits and not worry about our metabolism dropping.

Honestly, this is a great tool that has health benefits, can fit into a modern lifestyle, and can control the amount of food you eat.

Intermittent fasting can help you lose weight faster and keep it off because it's a method that controls your total food intake and prevents overeating, which automatically helps you lose weight.

And according to many gurus and traditional weight loss advice, eating 5-7 small meals a day is going to 'turn up your metabolism.'

The advice boils down to: If you eat more frequent meals, your body will have to increase its metabolic rate to break down that food. This is where the Thermic Effect of Food (TEF) comes in. The TEF is the energy required to digest food to get the calories.

The truth is though, it's just the total amount of food you eat that creates the thermic effect and calorie burn needed to break down and absorb your food. So it makes no difference whether you eat the same amount of food over 3 meals or 6 (46).

There was also the argument that small meals more often control blood sugars. This isn't shown in science. Studies show that people who eat fewer, larger meals have lower blood glucose levels on average (44). Less frequent eating has also been shown to improve satiety and reduce hunger compared to more frequent meals (45).

I took this into my own hands, and while I went through a 3-month stint of checking my blood glucose measurements an hour after every meal, I saw the exact same results. My blood sugars were lower when eating 4 meals a day compared to 7 meals a day.

Meal frequency per se has essentially no impact on the magnitude of weight or fat loss except for its effects on food intake. If a high meal frequency makes people eat more, they will gain weight because they are eating more. And if a high meal frequency makes people eat less, they will lose weight because they are eating less. But it's got nothing to do with stoking the metabolic fire or affecting metabolic rate on a day to day basis.

Most people find that they eat 3-4 meals a day, which could include one of them being a shake for ease. The beauty of having a window of time to eat is that by eating to the My Body Diet, you just eat the meals and foods that satisfy you.

Technically, having any proteins, vegetables, starches, fruits, amino acid drinks, or even fats is breaking your fast.

You will be learning to eat when hungry, and especially, why when starting with the first 14-Day Metabolic Switch Phase that I only want you to be focusing on eating the right foods and within the eating window set for you. I'll be giving you the right starting point and then being able to walk you through what changes you can make to fast-track your results.

If you're like me, you don't want to be eating really large meals that can just have you feeling like a stuffed chicken. I would much rather have a meal that has me satisfied for a few hours. And as I've already talked about in this book; the best diet plan is the one you'll stick to.

And when making changes, most often you don't want them to be dramatic, as your hunger patterns are established by your regular meal patterns that you have right now. This is why small changes will compound into great results.

The real truth boils down to that a hard and fast rule of "Fasting for 16 hours every day" is not going to work for many people.

This is where I want to empower you to have the right tools and knowledge to make it all fit into your life, and why the meal plans are designed to give you the best kickstart. And from there easy process can be made.

My Body Blends Intermittent Fasting for Fat-Loss Protocol:

Step 1: Set yourself an eating window.

Let's say, you choose to eat between 10am and 8pm.

Step 2: Have your first meal focused on a P-V-F meal.

Giving you a balanced blood sugar response with a strong injection of nutrition to have you thriving through the day.

Eat using the 80% principle, which is stop eating when you are 80% full. It takes time for your stomach to communicate to your brain that you're satisfied and this gives you an easy bumper so you don't overeat.

Step 3: Eat when you feel hungry.

Include meals in the My Body Diet.

Step 4: Enjoy your last meal at 8pm.

23
MAKING EATING FOR FAT LOSS SIMPLE

What's one of the biggest problems when it comes to you wanting to lose weight and really take care of your health…?

It's that it's made out to be so hard and confusing.

This was the main reason that I wanted to take the time to write this book for you, as any Google search on this topic is going to give you millions of search results, and so many of them are conflicting with polar opposite points of view. It leaves you scratching your head and having more questions than when you first started out. When I decided that I needed to lose weight and turn my life around, it was followed by endless hours of scrolling through websites trying to make sense of it all.

Then again, I was face-palmed with the fact that there are so many people trying to tell you to do different things. I remember early on in my career, I was publishing a monthly article in a fitness magazine. I was flicking through one issue and saw my article. Then, a few pages later, I saw another article recommending almost the exact opposite from what I had written about. It became clear to me then that I needed to focus on creating the simple to use, precise information that I knew was transforming my clients and members.

This is the problem when it comes to the debate of "clean eating" versus "flexible dieting." And this chapter has the main focus of following up after introducing you to the PFVC meal model, and making it really clear and simple when it comes to you answering the question of, "what foods do I eat?"

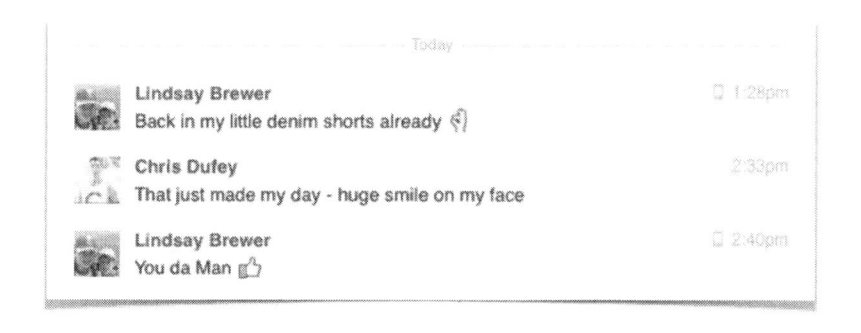

> Today
>
> **Lindsay Brewer** — 1:28pm
> Back in my little denim shorts already 🙋
>
> **Chris Dufey** — 2:33pm
> That just made my day - huge smile on my face
>
> **Lindsay Brewer** — 2:40pm
> You da Man 👍

Firstly, let's tackle clean eating and how the term has been used in so many different contexts; the term has basically become ambiguous.

One of the biggest battles you can have is cutting through the huge amount of conflicting information that is out there for when it comes you losing weight. This is one reason I highly respect Phil Graham. One of the best coaches, and thankfully, one that I've been able to learn so much from. It's easy to see that Phil has an incredible practical knowledge of what is needed when it comes to getting people in great shape, as one of the interviews we did together is named: How to Get Lean: The Proven Principles.

Much of what I have been able to piece together to gain a functional understanding and application has come about from Phil's impact on me. Because I've had to go through it first to easily understand what really matters for when it comes to you re-shaping your body, losing weight…

And, NOT: Getting caught up in the fuss of fads that just make it hard, confusing, and frustrating when wanting to look, feel, and function better each day.

What eating 'clean' foods is for one person, is something very different for someone else. Some people see the paleo diet as clean. Others see organic foods or mold-free foods as clean. Vegetarians will see one version, while others will see fruit or dairy as not clean. This is why I wanted to start you with the PFVC meal model and the basic shopping list and food choices that can become the foundation for your food choices. However, there is more to life than this food list. And more to what's 'optimal' for what is going to get you burning off the unwanted weight.

My own battle with "clean eating" started in Dubai. I was prepping for my first fitness model competition that was in London in 4 months' time. I had a very small list of select foods to stick to, and a piece of paper with the title "diet" that determined what I ate, when I ate, and how much of it I could eat. There is no doubt that the self-motivation to step on stage in front of the cameras and crowd in amazing shape got me through. I was carrying Tupperware containers of food around with me the whole time, and the majority of time eating cold food that was mainly chicken, green vegetables, and sweet potato. Then there was one moment that it all cracked.

Something triggered in me, and I don't even remember going to do it. But all I do remember is that I pretty much ate a whole jar of peanut butter. It was a food that I was 'not allowed' to eat, and when someone says don't think of a pink elephant… you think of a pink elephant. So this constant battling of thinking of what foods I had to stay away from, made me crave them even more. I have no doubt that it was not just the psychology, but also the physiological process of being deprived with a low-fat diet that made me want to go swimming in peanut butter.

You'll also learn in the next chapter how I ate so much Ben and Jerry's ice cream, it made me physically sick from the volume, and it made me purge it all back up. And I want to be open and transparent with you, opening up to show you that if you've had these battles before, It's all ok, but also, I don't ever want you to have to go through this again.

The big problem with restrictive eating is that it has a higher probability of binge eating. And this is exactly what I battled with, and unfortunately, I know first-hand through clients coming to me that other people were having these problems as well. It was interviewing Vera Tarman for the My Body Blends podcast when the mind-blowing truths came out. Just minutes into our interview, it became glaringly obvious that a very high majority of the 'health and fitness industry' has an eating disorder.

This is why I've designed the My Body Diet the way it is. As you need to burn more energy than you take in, but that DOES NOT mean you need to count calories to make this happen. Energy balance is the main factor for your body to be able to lose weight. However, there are factors of how many calories you consume and how many you burn based on your food choices.

This is why we start with a simple and highly effective plan that gets you choosing the right foods and eating until you're satisfied, and we need to look at foods and how they affect thermogenesis and satiety. For example, fiber improves satiety and thermogenesis.

Put simply, fiber refers to carbohydrates that cannot be digested by humans.

Insoluble fiber functions mostly as a 'bulking' agent and is also powerful in helping your digestion.

However… **Soluble fiber can have powerful effects on health and metabolism** (50).

We've previously talked about the huge importance of your gut health and the trillions of gut bacteria living in you right now. And it's the different species of gut flora that play important roles in your health, such as blood sugar control, weight management, immunity, and even brain function (51,52,53,54,55).

And this is where you need to feed your gut flora for them to stay healthy.

You do this by eating a mix of soluble and insoluble fiber, which has a prebiotic effect of having the beneficial results for health and bodyweight (56,57). The fiber passes through the digestive system mostly unchanged, eventually reaching your good bacteria, which can turn it into usable energy.

Soluble fiber is found in cucumbers, blueberries, beans, and nuts. Soluble fiber dissolves into a gel-like texture, helping to slow down your digestion. This helps you to feel full longer, which can help with weight control

Insoluble fiber, found in foods like dark green leafy vegetables, green beans, celery, and carrots does not dissolve and helps add bulk to your stool. This helps food to move through your digestive tract more quickly for healthy elimination

Another key difference between vegetables and fruits is the amount of water present. Water in a food makes a big difference. Because when water interacts with soluble fibers, the fiber will soak up that water like a sponge. This sponge effect is one of the major reason why soluble fibers work so well to blunt the return of hunger and stabilize blood sugar.

We've talked about the importance of controlling chronic inflammation and its powerful effects on your health and the ability to shape the body you want. Inflammation is a strong driver of disease, including heart disease, obesity, Alzheimer's, and metabolic syndrome (59,60,61). Gut bacteria has been shown to reduce inflammation (58). And one way that good bacteria does this is by producing short-chain, fatty acids that feed the cells in the colon.

How this starts to become powerful for you and burning off the unwanted weight is by lowering inflammation it has positive effects for fat loss via its effects on the hormone leptin (62,63,64). One of the important reasons for managing leptin is being able to control your appetite.

This is why we can have you eating less without trying.

One of the reasons I believe counting calories is not necessary is because we can set you up for "automatic fat loss" by controlling the amount of food you eat. Fiber will have the effect of reducing your appetite and having you feel satisfied between meals, and therefore, having you eat less.

A group of researchers from the University of Massachusetts Medical School zeroed in on fiber, since previous studies have shown it **can help people feel fuller, eat less,** and improve some metabolic markers like blood pressure, cholesterol levels, and blood sugar.

"By changing one thing, people in the fiber group were able to improve their diet and lose weight and improve their overall markers for metabolic syndrome," says study author Dr. Yunsheng Ma.

When it comes to diet guidelines, and how obesity, heart problems, and diabetes are so common, Ma says…

"Very few people reach the goals that are recommended. Asking them to focus on eating more of a certain food--rather than telling them what not to eat--may help people to think more positively about changes in their diet, and make the goals more achievable. From there, it might be easier to make the other changes. [Adding fiber] might be one new idea for how to get people to adhere to a diet."

And it's shown certain fibers, such as psyllium, glucomannan, guar gum, B-glucans, and pectins have the end results of having you feeling fuller for longer and significantly reducing appetite (65,66). It does this by becoming thicker and having a higher viscosity, forming a gel-like substance that sits in the gut (67).

Even with some science now showing that the **weight loss**

effect of sober can target belly fat that is also associated with metabolic disease (68).

The Best Ways to Get More Fiber

1. **Don't be a salad dodger…** Include veggies in each meal. Choosing between cooked and uncooked veggies will help get a broader range of nutrients.

Use the All You Can Eat Carb List to have plenty of great choices.

2. **Replace your bread and cereals with smarter carbs…** Especially when it comes to breakfast, you can make smarter choices that not only help you lose weight, but give you a boost in fiber intake.

A favorite of mine is a lean meat, such as chicken or steak, grilled with asparagus and green beans cooked in butter along with a handful of berries.

If you want a quicker option, the Low-Carb Breakfast Smoothie or Green Smoothie are great options to nourish yourself when you're on the go.

3. **Add a fiber supplement…** Taking 1 teaspoon to 1 tablespoon of a mixed fruit and vegetable fiber just before meals will help you feel more satisfied and burn more fat. This strategy works anytime you are worried about getting hungry or not eating a big enough meal. Many of our clients use fiber as a snack all by itself.

A good fiber supplement should have a high concentration of fruit and vegetable fibers such as lignin, pectin, gums, cellulose, and seeds. The fibers having the most research behind their action regarding fat loss include apple pectin and gums, such as guar and acacia.

In the supplements chapter that is to come, I walk you through what to look for with a good quality fiber supplement and how this can easily fit into your day to day plan.

How Protein Can Help You Lose Weight

There is a very good reason why protein is the first food that we put on our plate.

A high-protein intake boosts metabolism, reduces appetite, and changes several weight-regulating hormones (69,70,71). Protein can help you lose weight and belly fat, and it works via several different mechanisms.

A higher protein intake actually increases levels of the satiety (appetite-reducing) hormones GLP-1, peptide YY, and cholecystokinin, while reducing your levels of the hunger hormone ghrelin (72, 73, 74, 75,76). This leads to a major reduction in hunger and is the main reason protein helps you lose weight. It can automatically make you eat fewer calories.

Then there is also the factor that protein has a much higher Thermic Effect of Food (77).

As your body is going through the digestion process of breaking down the food to be able to absorb and assimilate it, the metabolism needs to burn energy to go through this process. And this is known as the Thermic Effect of Food (TEF).

Then on top of the increased TEF, your body will also burn

more calories during the day and even night (78,79). By making you burn more calories, high-protein diets have a "metabolic advantage" over diets that are lower in protein.

Protein can also reduce hunger through different pathways (80). Simply put, you end up eating fewer calories without having to count them or consciously control portions.

But then, there is also the factor that protein can help reduce cravings, late-night snacking, and obsessive thoughts of food.

This graph is from a study comparing a high-protein diet and a normal-protein diet in overweight men (81).

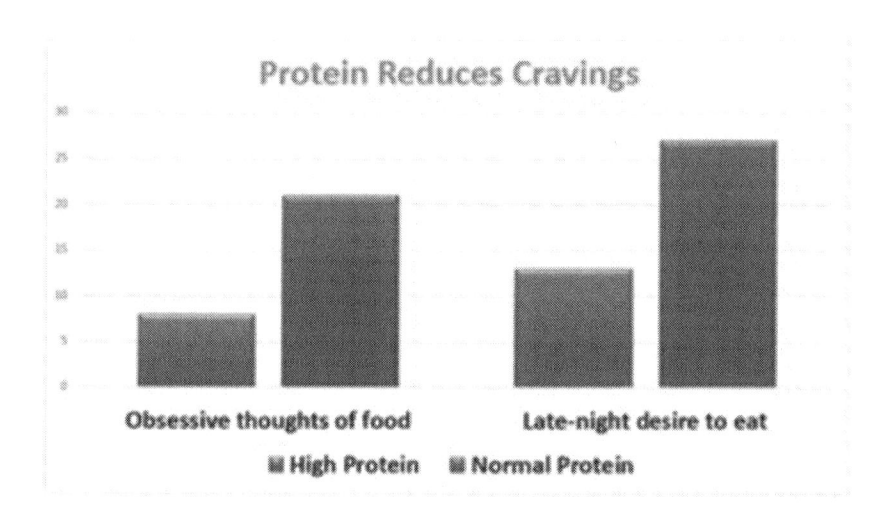

Protein Reduces Cravings

[Bar chart comparing High Protein and Normal Protein for Obsessive thoughts of food and Late-night desire to eat]

The high-protein group is the blue bar, while the normal-protein group is the red bar.

In this study, protein at 25% of calories reduced cravings by 60% and cut the desire for late-night snacking by half!

Protein works on both sides of the "calories in vs calories out" equation. It reduces calories in and boosts calories out.

For this reason, it is not surprising to see that high-protein diets lead to weight loss, even without intentionally restricting calories, portions, fat, or carbs (83, 84, 85).

Though remember, this entire plan isn't just about losing the unwanted weight quickly, it's also about keeping it off. Many people can go on "a diet" and lose weight, but most end up gaining the weight back (86). In one study, a small increase of protein reduced weight regained after weight loss by 50% (87).

This is why we include protein in each meal to spread your intake throughout the day.

Now that we've covered the importance of protein and getting enough fiber throughout each day, we can see that making the right food choices that makes this happen is simple.

On the flip side, the belief that if you just focus on eating a certain number of calories, or sticking to a certain number of proteins, fats, and carbs doesn't mesh with me. Mainly because there is a host of tracking and counting with calories and macronutrients. And I know that for the people who I write this book for, that is not what you want to do.

The reason that we have a quality first, over just focusing on quantity with your nutrition, is that you are going to have huge positive results, which come from you losing weight and lowering inflammation to having better clarity of mind and focus throughout the day.

The problem with a flexible dieting approach is the interpretation people have. For example, if I set the goal of eating 200 grams of carbohydrates in a day, I could eat ice cream every day, but that would take up a whopping amount of carbs and fats I could eat to still allow an energy deficit.

Not only would I be losing out on the micronutrients I could get from eating whole, nutrient-dense foods that give me the same carbs and fats, it's much more likely that I'll be hungrier throughout the day. And the impact on gut health, and the psychology behind 'junk food' makes it clear to me, that ice cream isn't an everyday food for me.

Technically, you could live off Pop Tarts, protein shakes, and fiber supplements and still hit your macronutrient targets. This is not a great long-term strategy for your body's composition or health.

And this is where it becomes a balancing act. And most importantly, why I wrote this for you, is to show you that no one, no, not me, not any guru, not any book, can give you the precise set of foods and amounts for you to eat to lose the weight and happily live your life.

This is why we designed the My Body Diet to start the Metabolic Priming Phase, and have the important steps after it. Because it gives you back the power. You have the power to make the smart and impactful choices. As Jade Teta puts so well, you become the detective for what works for you.

Your weight is determined by how many calories you consume and expend (92,93). However, where you get those calories also matters.

Your macronutrient intake and food choices also play a major role in your ability to lose fat, gain muscle, stay full, stay healthy, perform well physically, and just about everything else.

Food quality and quantity are completely intertwined and impossible to separate.

Controlling your portions is important for making sure you get enough nutrition, as well as making sure you don't overindulge. Likewise, eating more filling and nutritious food helps you control your portion sizes by keeping you satiated and well-nourished with fewer calories (94,95).

24
REFUEL MEALS AND THE DEATH OF CHEATING

Now we're answering the all too popular question…

Cheat meals!

Should I have cheat meals?

What do I eat?

How much do I eat?

Do you ever have cheat meals, Chris?

And this first starts with.

If you think, steak, potatoes, and mango sticky rice are 'cheat foods'… You're on the wrong diet.

These are some of the foods I've eaten this week.

If you are trying to follow a "zero tolerance" diet, where you are trying to go for weeks to months without enjoying your favorite foods, often binging and suffering from 'fat re-bound' where you gain all the weight you lost over several months (in just days to weeks), it can become a big problem for you.

And this is where I have good news and bad news for you.

The bad news is:

With many diet plans telling you that cheat meals and cheat days are important for you. The real truth that's come from learning from the experts and seeing the first-hand results with clients all around the world: Is that all too often, cheat meals are causing you harm.

The good news is:

I've given up cheat meals… and now have members happily following simple meal plans that include their favorite foods. They lose weight faster and enjoy the process.

And that's what I want to share with you now.

Firstly, let's cover why I DON'T love "cheat meals"…

Giving you the right plan that prevents you from feeling deprived, boosting your metabolism, and setting you up for success is why I created the My Body Diet. And feeling overly deprived, only to finally cave into the temptations that have been haunting you, has been shown to result in binge eating, and with you overeating (with foods that can only cause harm to your digestive health). You will soon see that there is a strong connection in how your body and brain regulates the food you eat, and what foods you're going to continue to crave.

No!

This does not mean that we strike all of our favorite foods from your allowable foods. In fact, it's the opposite. We are going to use refuel meals to have a strong body and brain, and a positive impact to you burning off the unwanted weight and not feeling deprived.

I do use "refuel meals." As in eating more carbs or calories than usual in one day or in a meal. These might be called <u>healthy</u> cheats, but you're going to find how to "have your cake and eat it too" in this chapter.

The common belief that cheat meals have people quickly turn to a binge-eating fest of the foods that are being deprived of when "on the diet." It's causing harm, as you'll soon discover.

An important concept is "starvation mode," and how this is mostly a myth. As we've already covered, you don't need to eat small frequent meals to "stoke your metabolic fire." And we've found that fasting has numerous benefits and can be used easily within a realistic lifestyle.

The belief of starvation mode and cheat meals I see has mainly come from the bodybuilding world. And how, when on a long dieting phase to prepare for a physique show and to reach low depths of body fat, you do need to use tools such as refeeding with meals that boost carbs and calories.

However, most people are not preparing for a bodybuilding show, or in super low depths of body fat that there is a physiological need for a burst of food.

On the flip side, I have to be 100% realistic, and there are physiologic and psychological benefits to refuel meals.

There is one thing we need to cover before we jump into why refuel meals are going to change your body. And it's that there is no doubt that the power of words plays a big role in how we act and feel.

A research study divided people into two groups: one group was told that each time they were faced with a temptation, they would tell themselves "I CAN'T do X." For example, when tempted with ice cream, they would say, "I can't eat ice cream." The second group was told to say, "I DON'T do X." For example, when tempted with ice cream, they would say, "I don't eat ice cream."

As each student walked out of the room and handed in their answer sheet, they were offered a complimentary treat. The student could choose between a chocolate candy bar or a health bar. As the student walked away, the researcher would mark their snack choice on the answer sheet.

The students who told themselves "I can't eat X" chose to eat the chocolate candy bar 61% of the time. Meanwhile, the students who told themselves "I don't eat X" chose to eat the chocolate candy bars only 36% of the time. (91)

Since doing away with 'cheat meals,' I've been able to easily stay lean all year round, and my relationship with food is healthier than ever. And it was soon after noticing the changes in myself, that I passed this onto clients for them only come back weeks after, already noticing a physical and psychological difference.

And this is why I want to ask you…

Does this sound familiar:

- If you eat all your veggies, then you can eat dessert.
- If you go for a run, then you can splurge later because you deserved it.
- If it's your cheat meal, you can eat whatever you want.

Each of these sets you up for failure.

Have you fallen off the wagon before, only to spiral out of control and struggle to get back on.

It all starts with; "I'll have some pizza… and a glass of wine… yeah ok, I'll have the ice cream… Oh, you're having the brownie. Sure, I'll have one too."

And it continues on and on. One meal turns into a whole day, turns into a whole weekend, as you say to yourself.

"I'll start on Monday."

One meal has turned into a splurge fest that can not only damage you and your previous weeks of hard work, it also makes it harder for you to keep moving forward.

This brings us to the psychological force known as the 'compensation effect.' The compensation effect refers to the tendency for people to assume they accumulate moral capital. We use good deeds to balance out bad deeds, or alternately, we give ourselves breaks from goodness, like a piece of chocolate after a week of salads. This makes people more inclined to do bad things under the guise of "I'm a good person" or "It's just this one thing."

But even more interesting is cognitive dissonance. Cognitive dissonance is the discomfort humans feel when they hold two contradictory opinions or their behavior is inconsistent with their beliefs. It's one of the strongest psychological forces driving human behavior. When people who feel they are good do bad things, cognitive dissonance makes them ignore this behavior because they can't tolerate the inconsistency between their behavior and their beliefs. People high with emotional intelligence suffer less from cognitive dissonance.

This is why I want you to use refuel meals. As it makes the diet more enjoyable and gives you both body and brain benefits.

However, that being said, how you use refuel meals matters. And why I've seen a huge number of people use 'cheat meals' the wrong way, and seen them create a pile of frustration and fat gain.

For example, the biggest mistakes I see people make are…

- 'Cheating' too frequently.
- Eating too much in their cheat meals.
- Indulging in cheat days, not meals.
- Eating too much dietary fat.
- Drinking too much alcohol.

And this starts with your brain…

How Your Brain Eats

Your brain, spinal cord, and nerves intertwine to be able to communicate with your digestive organs. Let's say you're about to eat an ice cream cone. The notion and image of that ice cream occur in the higher center of the brain – the cerebral cortex. From there, information is relayed electrochemically to the limbic system, which is considered the "lower" portion of the brain. The limbic system regulates emotions and key physiological functions, such as hunger, thirst, temperature, sex drive, heart rate, and blood pressure. Within the limbic system, is a pea-sized collection of tissues known as the hypothalamus, which integrates the activities of the mind with the biology of the body. In other words, it takes sensory, emotional, and thought input and transduces this information into physiological responses.

"Cheat meals" implies you're doing something wrong and brings about guilt, and there should be no guilt when it comes to eating food. When you're only eating your favorite mango sticky rice (ok, it's one of my favorites), then you're cheating. You're creating a dichotomy and seeing it as a "good" food versus "bad" food.

And this sets you up to see yourself as good when you only eat the good foods, and bad for when you eat the bad foods.

And no, I don't think this is just semantics.

If the ice cream is your favorite flavor – say, chocolate – and you consume it with a full measure of delight, the hypothalamus will modulate this positive input by sending activation signals via parasympathetic nerve fibers to the salivary glands, esophagus, stomach, intestines, pancreas, liver, and gallbladder. Digestion will be stimulated, and you'll have a fuller metabolic breakdown of the ice cream while burning its calories more efficiently.

If you're feeling guilty about eating the ice cream or judging yourself for eating it, the hypothalamus will take this negative input and send signals down the sympathetic fibers of the autonomic nervous system. This initiates inhibitory responses in the digestive organs, which means you'll be eating your ice cream but not fully metabolizing it. It may stay in your digestive system longer, which can diminish your population of healthy gut bacteria and increase the release of toxic by-products into the bloodstream. Furthermore, inhibitory signals in the nervous system can decrease your calorie-burning efficiency via increased insulin and cortisol, which would cause you to store more of your guilt-infused ice cream as body fat. So the thoughts you think about the food you eat instantly become reality in your body via the central nervous system.

This is where I found myself being a big wimp…

Feeling guilty during and/or after a meal means you're not getting the enjoyment and satisfaction of it.

Bloated, guilty, and miserable was how I was commonly feeling after cheat meals. When the thought hit me - "what's the point?"

The cheat meal may give you some pleasure while you are eating it, but it can have you feeling miserable afterward.

The secret is moderation and portion control. And we can set you up to have these two working for you when following the My Body Diet and using the Refuel Meal Guide I have for you below.

But there come the cold hard facts about junk food… and why the 'clean eaters' have it both right and wrong.

I wanted to wait until now to share with you the surprising truth behind why we crave junk food.

We know 'junk food' is unhealthy for us. And it's not going to be the best choice for us to get in the body shape we want.

But, even with us knowing this… why do we keep doing it? (At least, until now.)

To answer this question, I discovered Steven Witherly, a food scientist who wrote the fantastic Why Humans Love Junk Food. He's one of the world's top experts from having the experience of over 20 years studying what makes certain foods more addictive (and tasty) than others.

There are two factors that make junk food a trap for a strong temptation.

The actual sensation of eating food is a strong component that I also learned from Marc David with the first interview we did for the My Body Blends Podcast. The sensation of eating includes what it tastes like (sweet, salty, sourness, bitterness, and umami), what it smells like, and also, how it feels in your mouth.

Then there is also <u>orosensation,</u> which is why food companies will spend millions of dollars finding the most pleasurable crunch of a potato chip, or how a soft drink will dance on your tongue for example.

The second half is the makeup of the food. The blend of proteins, fats, and carbohydrates it has. And this is where food manufacturers are looking for a perfect combination of salt, sugar, and fat that excites your brain and gets you to crave more of it.

Food engineers can use dynamic contrasts like a creme Brule or an Oreo cookie, or create the right salivary response that makes sauces and ice creams create a pleasurable response with the brain.

A fantastic example of this is one that Robb Wolfe highlights in his book, Wired To Eat. When reading this, I had to laugh for two reasons. One being that I remember watching the exact episode of Man vs Food that Robb refers to. And the other was because I know I have fallen prey to this problem.

In this one particular episode of Man vs Food, Adam Rickman takes on the challenge of eating a kitchen sink full of ice cream. Now, we've already talked about my love of ice cream, so the first thought when the episode started was, how awesome is this. Though it quickly turned into compassionate disgust as I watched Adam Rickman quickly hit a wall as he tried to eat through this gigantic portion of ice cream.

Robb highlighted so brilliantly that typical thinking that has us believe that because Adam Rickman is eating such a sheer volume of food and calories, his body is simply not going to allow any more to go in.

But Adam Rickman does something very interesting. He orders a side of extra crispy, extra salty french fries. And by alternating between the french fries and ice cream, he is able to eat the entire kitchen sink of ice cream. Which sounds absurd, as he added MORE food and many, many more calories to get through the challenge. But this highlights that there is more going on than just food volume and calories that have us eating the foods and amounts we do.

The difference in food texture, palatability, taste, and sensation on the brain from the french fries and ice cream allows us to bypass the switch that tells the brain that you're full and satisfied.

This can also be seen for when you go to a buffet. You can eat a big dinner and be sitting there with your belt unbuckled, rubbing your stomach like a genie is about to pop out and be satisfied from all he food. However, if dessert is offered soon after, all of a sudden, you have room for the sweet dish that's on offer.

There is also the calorie density problem with junk foods, as they are designed to tell your brain that you're getting nutrition, but not to fill you up.

Then there is what's called 'rapid food meltdown' and the 'vanishing calorie density.'

In his best-selling book, Salt Sugar Fat, author Michael Moss describes a conversation with Witherly that perfectly explains vanishing caloric density…

I brought him two shopping bags filled with a variety of chips to taste. He zeroed right in on the Cheetos. "This," Witherly said, "is one of the most marvelously constructed foods on the planet in terms of pure pleasure." He ticked off a dozen attributes of the Cheetos that make the brain say more. But the one he focused on most was the puff's uncanny ability to melt in the mouth. "It's called vanishing caloric density," Witherly said. "If something melts down quickly, your brain thinks that there's no calories in it … you can just keep eating it forever."

Lastly, there is the factor of what memories you have of past eating experiences.

There's no doubt that I love cookies and ice cream, because as a child, I had great times that involved me eating those foods.

What's the result of all of this… You can easily overeat.

And this is where the good news is that research shows the less junk food you eat, the less you crave it. And it's exactly what I've found myself and with countless clients.

Now knowing this, we can easily set up the plan and your environment to help you not fall into the junk food trap, for when you don't want to be eating it.

The Real Benefits of a Refuel Meal Done Right

There are two main reasons that we want to enjoy our favorite foods and have refuel meals.

Firstly, let's look at the physiological reasons.

Long-term dieting can decrease your metabolic rate and important metabolic hormones, such as leptin and thyroid. Studies have shown that leptin levels can decrease by up to 39% in 4 days and up to 54% in a week (88,89,90).

Increasing your leptin, liver glycogen, testosterone, Growth Hormone, and thyroid levels as well as lowering your cortisol levels, can have you reigniting your fat burning metabolism.

This directly impacts your body's ability to burn through body fat and can increase hunger.

Leptin is synthesized in adipose tissue (fat cells) so the smaller the fat cells are, the lower the leptin production. Which, in turn, increases hunger and lowers your energy expenditure levels. And it's low-carbohydrate nutrition that seems to affect leptin levels the most.

Now, a lower carb, or what we call a smarter carb approach, is what best suits the vast majority of people. And that includes me! Which is why many people, when following the traditional diet advice, will further reduce their calories, cut their carbs back even more, and increase their exercise by large amounts when they hit a fat-loss plateau.

Then there is the psychological reason I want you to eat your favorite foods and enjoy refuel meals.

And it's my belief that adherence to a plan is the single most important factor for long-term success. This is why the My Body Diet has been designed the way it has. To give you an easy start with simple steps moving forward. Totally understanding that you are your own unique person and lifestyle, and it has to match that.

The first question is; What are your goals?

For me, I want to look, feel, and function phenomenally each and every day.

The fact that I am the face of my business and brand isn't that much of a strong motivator. As I know, deep down, I have to just be open and honest about who I am.

If you are wanting to lose 5-10 pounds, to feel confident in your body, and be able to be the best version of you, then you are going to be able to use refuel meals in a smart way having the four guiding principles I show you below help you make the right decisions.

If you want to get into low depths of body fat and even compete as a physique model or bodybuilder, then you need to use more extreme measures and tools.

The second question to ask yourself is; Are you feeling deprived?

On a physiological side. Are you feeling flat, your muscle bellies are flat, your energy levels have plummeted, your sex drive is at rock bottom, you're struggling to get a 'pump' in the gym. These are all factors that can show that it's time to refuel your body.

On the psychological side. Are you feeling deprived and are your cravings and urges are getting worse and worse?

If you're going through each day and just trying to grit your teeth and battle through the urges, then it's time to make some adjustments.

Let's look at the lifetime changes we can start to make now. And how this is truly going to become a lifestyle for you that you can happily go through each day where the side effect is less body fat and a better performing body.

Thirdly. How often are you going to have your refuel meals?

After the initial 14-Day Metabolic Switch, we use an easy rule of thumb refuel meal once a week.

4 meals day would equal 14 meals - so one of those can be your refuel meal

Now, I'm also going to add in here the difference for if someone wants to get into low depths of body fat. There is no specific point that a refuel is needed. The factors of your body's fat levels, training volume and frequency, the amount of muscle mass you have, and how you're feeling and performing all come into the equation.

This is where a really experienced and proven coach is worth their weight in gold.

The next question is: How motivated are you?

When I was prepping for a fitness model show, it was a highly motivated goal I had set myself. It's why I would get up in the early hours of the morning to go and train before seeing clients. It's why

I would eat the same few meals over and over. Not really bothered at all about it.

Now, I'm a dad of two beautiful girls, running two businesses and it's not my goal to be super lean. I can live a balance of being in the shape I want and have my brain performance optimized so I can produce the best work I can and enjoy the fruits of life I choose.

If you're going through a fat-loss phase, and have set out to achieve great results, then yes, absolutely, I think you should be focused, and you can use that motivation to make the right decisions that get you the results you want.

Lastly, there is the question. How much should you eat?

Just two weeks out from the last time I competed as a fitness model, I had a refuel day where I needed to hit 1000 grams of carbohydrates that day. I thought it was going to be fantastic, but the night finished off with me ripping open a bag of confectionary lollies to get the last 150 grams of carbs in me.

I was bloated from the full day of eating mountains of rice and gluten-free cereal. Going to bed that night, I didn't know if I had done the right thing. However, I woke up leaner, and with veins running across my entire body that it kind of disgusted my wife, Lauren.

The leaner you are, the more carbs you will need by rule of thumb, and the more often you will need refuel meals.

Now you can use these four principles to make refuel meals work for you…

1. Eat protein and vegetables first in your meal. Sit down and enjoy a meal that is rich in protein and vegetables. I've gone in-depth with the importance of protein and fiber, but this is also going to keep you full – it's going to save you going crazy, and also help blunt the blood sugar response.

2. If you want to go for seconds… Have another protein and veg meal first.

When you've had your refuel meal, and enjoyed your favorite foods, and the carbs working its way through your tummy, you may want to eat more. And that's perfectly fine.

The one principle we have in place for this is that you just eat another protein and vegetable meal first, before diving into more carbs or dessert.

This saves you from binge-eating on the carbs and sugar.

3. Plan your refuel meal ahead of time. It can all go to ruin if you suddenly say, "screw it, let's do it."

Because one thing leads to another, and you're sitting down having devoured piles of food as you didn't really think about what was going on. Decide on what you're going to enjoy, and where you're going to enjoy it.

4. Enjoy it! Food is something surrounding all major celebrations. Birthdays, Christmas, Weddings… they all involve food. Both sides of my family have food heavily centered around family traditions.

My grandmothers would take great pride in being able to feed and nourish their families with great meals. And food is a social thing!

So go and enjoy it with others you love and love to be around.

25
WORKOUT LESS FOR FASTER RESULTS

There is no doubt that nutrition makes up a large chunk of what is going to bring about your results. And there's a good chance you've heard the phrase "abs are made in the kitchen." While it's cute, many health and fitness people debate the ratio of importance of nutrition to achieving fat loss, the commonly regurgitated number is it's 70% diet and 30% training.

Again, it's all cute to spit a number like that out, but let's just cut to the chase and say they are 100% equal, and we're going to make smarter decisions with both from now on. Why I didn't want to write a 'diet book' is because it goes so much farther than just diet to achieve the physique and health you want.

That's why the second pillar to results is; Moving every day.

This is where, when I asked a better question such as, "What is the right exercise and training I should be doing?" We get a much more effective way to train to create fast and long-lasting body transformations.

We've already covered that the "eat less and move more" advice for weight loss is severely flawed in relation to your eating. And when the approach of just trying to burn more calories with exercise is applied, it can get you sidetracked. As the majority of the energy you are going to burn through in a day is not through exercise, it's through your resting metabolic rate (RMR). And when you look at how many calories you can burn in one training session, going for a 45-minute run will burn through more calories in that time frame compared to 45 minutes of traditional weight training. However, the huge difference is in the effect you have after the training session, which makes all the difference (I will show you why and how just below).

Just before we dive into what the best training and movement is to have you looking and feeling phenomenal, let's gently bring the focus back to what your goal is. As I don't blame everyone right now that are still fixated that losing scale weight is the goal. This is why there are so many people still "scared" of so many of the training programs that are excellent for accelerating fat loss. Let's start from the assumption that the primary goal of dieting is to lose fat while maintaining muscle mass (or at least minimizing the loss of muscle that often occurs).

Now let's look at the type of training I recommend, and also cover why I suggest some forms of training or movement that other health professionals wrongly avoid.

Before we dive into the type of training I recommend and also cover why I suggest some forms of training or movement that other health professionals wrongly avoid, let's stamp out some of the nonsense many fitness professionals are preaching at the moment. And that is; running is causing weight gain problems. They are preaching that going out and doing low-intensity cardio is actually causing you to gain weight. And this is where we need to see the difference of "it doesn't work" to "there's a better way." One of the most important factors is when it comes to training, you are doing something. If we get you going from the couch to going for a job, a bike ride, or even a Zumba class, then, fantastic, this is a positive step for your health. And so many weight loss programs miss the point that there does have to be an element that you enjoy what you do for you to be able to keep it up and, therefore, get your rewards for it.

When we look at "there's a better way" to have you accelerating fat loss, then we can jump into this next section to clearly see what is going to be the most effective approach.

Reading through a very in-depth article on the metabolism of carbohydrates and their optimal use for fat loss, was when I got to the bottom of the article, I first saw the name, Scott Stevenson.

I was so impressed by the article and quality of information, I immediately started to search for who Scott was, and how I best could contact him. I knew that I had to interview him and learn from the immense wealth of information he had.

Not long after, I interviewed Scott for the very first time and recently discovered that he is the founder of Fortitude Training. He's been very generous in sharing the ins and outs of how to best structure workout routines, and how the interplay of nutrition and training need to be best designed.

I say with full thanks, that what I've learned from Scott has hugely impacted the way I design programs.

This is where we use a mix of methods, each with their own uniqueness and need to get your body moving and responding in the right way. We combine Metabolic Resistance Training (MRT) with Metabolic Conditioning (Met Con), along with our Yin Movements. These names are arbitrary, I didn't make them up, and I'm sure if you used these three names with other people, you'd get a different response to what they are. However, to keep it simple, I'll walk you through what these are, so we can understand the exact definition.

26

METABOLIC RESISTANCE TRAINING

Metabolic Resistance Training

How can you walk into your next workout –

And use one of the most popular fat-loss training methods:

Metabolic Resistance Training.

This is the exact training that has dominated the workout programs for fat loss. And there's good reason:

- **You're going to save time.** These workouts can halve your training time.
- **You're going produce higher lactate** and, therefore, more Growth Hormone that speeds up your fat loss.

- **You're going to be able to boost your metabolism** for up 38 hours after each workout.

But before we dive into Metabolic Resistance Training, let me share with you a secret I haven't exposed before.

I got stuck at a point of around 10-12% body fat, and where I couldn't lose any more weight.

I was cutting my carbs, eating less food, and training every day. But each week when I checked in for results, all I found was I was losing motivation from a lack of results.

Then I came across John Romaniello. I quickly got on board his Final Phase Fat-Loss program. And this is where I first came across Metabolic Resistance Training, and discovered that I had been wasting a whole lot of time and effort with the wrong training methods.

These workouts I have for you can fit into your busy days with ease, plus, most members find them more fun.

We use the key principles that make up the most efficient way to exercise to burn fat with your training when designing the Metabolic Resistance Training (MRT) style workouts.

I think we've hammered home that the "eat less and move more" advice for weight loss is severely flawed, and when the approach of just trying to burn more calories with exercise is applied can get you sidetracked.

The majority of the energy you are going to burn through in a day is not through exercise, it's through your resting metabolic rate

(RMR). And when you look at how many calories you can burn in one training session, going for a 45-minute run will burn through more calories in that time frame compared to 45 minutes of traditional weight training. However, it is the huge difference in the effect you have after the training session that makes all the difference.

The overall training effect of Metabolic Resistance Training is a greater metabolic disturbance in the body's physiology, which in turn, can elevate your caloric expenditure for a greater period of time following your workout. Also, the term Metabolic Resistance Training is broad, and depending on who's using it will mean different things. In the context for us and the training programs I'm giving you, it can vary from body weight workouts, to heavy weight training. But all have the focus on body composition changes to elect fat loss and lean muscle gain.

Hala Rambie, a Romanian exercise scientist, found that the lactic acid pathway was more effective for fat loss than the aerobic pathway. Ramble determined that the high blood lactic levels decreased blood pH levels, which in turn, increases production of Growth Hormone.

To do this most effectively, we increase the time under tension, but also, importantly, we keep the intensity of the exercises higher. And this is done by using heavier weights, and especially in relation to the old-dogmatic approach of high reps, such as 20 reps per set, which forces the trainee to use light weights.

The increased time under tension, intensity, and short rest intervals lead to an increased production of lactate, and an increase in lactate leads to dramatic increases in Growth Hormone, thus resulting in very significant losses of body fat.

Growth Hormone accelerates lipolysis, the breakdown of lipids, and involves hydrolysis of triglycerides into glycerol and free fatty acids, and impaired secretion of human growth hormone leads to loss of lipolytic effect. This is why the smarter workouts I'm going to be taking you through have a profound effect on your fat loss.

Also, with these MRT workouts, you are going to have a jump in adrenaline. And this is an important hormone that helps with the mobilization of fatty acids. This means that you're going to be opening the floodgates so that your body is actually able to burn fat for fuel. In comparison, traditional weight loss workouts can just be using the energy pathways that are not effective in actually tapping into fat to be burned.

One of the leading experts, when it comes to effective and efficient training, is Nick Tumminello. Just some of the brilliance behind what Nick does is break down hard science and topics that can leave your head-spinning into easy to understand and use advice.

This is a sign of someone truly being a master of their craft. The very first interview we held together was on "Breaking down the fitness fads (so you can use what works)." And he has had a direct impact on the design and structure of the training programs so that you can have the best results without wasting your time and energy.

Plus, you will have a heightened metabolism that combines with the increase in metabolic hormones to create an 'afterburn' effect. Excess post-exercise oxygen consumption (EPOC) is the measurable increase of oxygen intake following strenuous exercise that's intended to erase the 'oxygen deficit.' This is where you can have an increase in calorie and fat burning for up to 38 hours after each workout (37).

You will see in the example training workouts below, the reason we pair exercises back to back is so one muscle is able to recover, while the opposing muscle is working. This way, you can get more work done inside each training session.

The other major benefit of this style of training is the increase in insulin sensitivity. Weight training is one of the best forms of 'glucose disposal' so that you are pushing your muscles to take in nutrients and especially glucose from carbohydrates you eat, and avoiding it being stored in fat cells.

Along with the positive changes in metabolic hormones, the increase in calorie and fat burning for up to 38 hours after each workout, and increased insulin sensitivity the lifestyle benefits that many of my client's love, is that your workouts are going to be shorter, and you won't be going to the gym as often.

This is because the frequency of training is not the typical bodybuilding split of weight training hitting one muscle group per week. Instead, you will be able to train each muscle more often. So, you have your chest on Mondays, quads on Tuesdays and so on… Even by only weight training three times a week, you will be able to have a high enough stimulus to produce the body-changing results you're looking for.

With the programs that you get here in the book and also in the Free Download section, you will be able to have a training program that suits the number of workouts you can happily fit into your lifestyle.

27
LESS RUNNING MORE MET CON CARDIO FOR FAT LOSS

It's time to kill off the myth of the "fat burning zone."

All too often, you will still see cardio machines showing graphs and numbers that separate "fat burning" and "cardiovascular training."

This idea that if you keep your heart rate in the 'fat burning zone,' which is roughly 55% to 65% of your maximum heart rate, is that you will be able to burn more fat than at higher levels of exercise intensity. This came about because the way your body uses energy is pulling from either fat or glycogen stores. At lower levels of exercise intensity, you will be burning a relatively higher percentage of fat compared to glycogen. At 50% of your max heart rate, your body burns a ratio of 60% fat to 40% glycogen. At 75% of your max heart rate, the ratio is 35% to 65% (41).

Though, if you exercise for 30 minutes at low intensity (50% of your max), you will burn roughly a total of 200 calories, 120 of those calories from fat. If you exercise at a higher intensity (75% of your max), you will burn 400 calories, in which 140 will come from fat.

So yes, even though the ratio is higher fat to glycogen at lower levels of intensity, because you will be burning more energy in total at a higher intensity, you will still be burning more fat. Plus, there are two other benefits. The first is that burning glycogen is a good thing, and also, the EPOC effect that I touched on before will come about from higher intensity exercise.

You're going to see that one of the most popular methods for weight loss, which is going out for a medium intensity run, is one of the worst ways in which to burn off body fat. And also, why, for many, it's a combination of high-intensity exercise and low-intensity exercise, such as walking, that can be a potent plan for burning off stubborn fat.

Craig Ballantyne did such an amazing job that I've had him on the show three times already. Each time, delving deeper and deeper into topics and unveiling the real truth to what brings about results. Craig Ballantyne, the creator of Turbulence Training, and also, co-author of The Great Cardio Myth, reveals so well why cardio won't get you slim, strong, or healthy - and the new high-intensity training plan will.

The Metabolic Conditioning (Met Con) style workouts that I will be giving you in the workout section, and also the Bonus

Downloads you get free access to, are designed to be short and effective.

The dramatic benefit of Met Con is supported by several studies, such as those conducted by researchers at Laval University, Baylor College of Medicine, and University of New South Wales. These have all shown that shorter, high-intensity cardio sessions result in greater fat loss over time than longer low-intensity sessions (40).

The scientists have shown that the positive factors of Met Con style training are:
- Increased resting metabolic rate for more than 24 hours after exercise.
- Improved insulin sensitivity in the muscle.
- High levels of fat oxidization in the muscles.
- Spike in Growth Hormone and catecholamine (such as Epinephrine) that aid in fat loss and induce fat mobilization.

How Often Should I Do This?

Many people are shocked to learn how little time I, and what I tell my clients, spend in the gym training each week. Unfortunately, the quantity over quality continues through the myths of weight loss. Where so many are caught up with trying to do more and go harder with their exercise, they are losing sight of what is a smarter approach that will give the stimulus needed for the body to change.

The 'maximum effect dose' can quickly come into play when people are steadfast on trying to lose as much fat and getting as lean as possible. Which I totally understand, and I certainly fell into this trap for many years.

For far too long, I was trying to get as many high-intensity weight and cardio sessions in per week, often doing 'double days' where I would weight train in the evening and come back in the afternoon to do either another weight or a sprint session. Now when programmed right and ensuring optimal recovery, this can be done effectively. And that's why I'm going to walk you through how to easily improve your recovery, and how to have the right balance of what you need to be doing.

The starting base of "how many times should I train each week?" is a minimum of four sessions per week. I've found over the years, this level has proven far superior than 2 or 3 workouts per week. But it's also the 'type' of workouts that, when following the plans I give you here, will be accelerating your results.

What I want you to be able to decide is, "how many workouts can you fit into your lifestyle?" If you decide that you can work out five times a week, then four MRT workouts and one cardio based workout are perfectly fine.

Metabolic Resistance workouts can vary from three to five times a week. Where Metabolic Conditioning workouts can vary from 1-2 times a week. But it's also why I'm about to walk you through the importance of 'Yin' movement, and even why walking can be a potent part of your fat burning plan.

Example Workout Frequency		
Training Days Per Week	MRT Sessions	Met Con Sessions
3	3	0
4	3	1
5	4	1
6	4	2

Again, this is where the power lies in your hands. It depends on what you what you enjoy, but the graph above gives a very common, and preferred split, of how many workouts you do in what style, depending on how many times a week you can train.

But, before we do, let's cover an important question that comes up, and then we can ensure you have the right answers surrounding your hunger and training.

How Your Training Affects Your Hunger

The question of "If I start training, won't I just become hungrier and eat more?" comes up often, and it's a good question. Though the positive benefits are another great reason to be moving your body the right way.

This seems to be related to increased levels of various gut

hormones involved in signaling fullness, also, exercise can increase leptin transport into the brain (other studies suggest that long-term aerobic activity may improve leptin sensitivity which is good given that obesity is generally associated with leptin resistance in the brain). There may still be as of yet undiscovered mechanisms for exercise to impact hunger/appetite.

Other work suggests that even if exercise can increase hunger, any increase in food intake tends to be less than the energy burned during the activity itself; that is exercise still has an overall benefit. It's worth mentioning that, even here, there tends to be a large degree of individuality, some people compensate for the energy expenditure of activity better than others, and this may be part of what contributes to individual differences in results.

Beginners often seem to get a slight increase in hunger following activity, at least in the first few weeks of training. I suspect this is due to their general over-reliance on glucose for fuel (falling blood glucose being one of many stimuli for hunger). At about the week four mark, as their bodies start to get the first adaptation to training and start to use more fat for fuel, this effect generally goes away.

Even beyond that, exercise has continued to show the great benefits with regards to health and overall body fat reduction. And even more so, the positive impact on weight loss maintenance, which brings us back around to the importance of being able to keep the weight off and not have the yo-yo dieting problem.

This metabolic type training will generate a higher calorie burn and with the 'afterburn' effect lasting up to 38 hours after each workout, along with the glycogen depletion and insulin sensitivity that further enhances fat loss, and then again, with the positive hormonal response.

28
THE YIN TO YOUR YANG YOUR WORKOUT PLAN

At about six years into my fitness career, I was more motivated than ever to up-skill myself to give my clients what was needed for the best results. And at one point, I was completing a sports massage therapist course, as this was a prerequisite for me to then study and become qualified as an Active Release Technique (ART) therapist.

This meant that a usual day had me waking at 4:30am, to then see clients from 6:00am to mid-afternoon, and then jumping straight into the car and driving for 45 minutes to have two hours of sports massage therapy class. At the same time, I was still training six days a week, which was a mix of heavy weight training and High-Intensity Interval Training.

It all came to a crashing halt as my energy, libido, self-drive, and general happiness and wellbeing dropped to rock bottom. I went to see a Functional Medicine Doctor that I had seen before and was referring clients to, to receive the much-needed slap in the face of the truth that I was wearing myself out.

We can all become "busy" in our modern lifestyle. And now, I've learned to take the word 'busy' out of my vocabulary, and I can't complain to anybody about me being too busy. As Tim Ferriss says so well, "busyness is a form of laziness, and lack of priorities." And when it comes to your exercise and training, it's NOT all about going as hard as you can every day and in every training session.

In Traditional Chinese Medicine, the underlying principles of good health are believed to come from a balance of Yin and Yang. For a long time, I thought it was just a need to work harder and do more to force results. It was all yang focused, with more training sessions, more sets, more weight, more interval training, and being stricter with diet and cutting foods down even more.

Well, this doesn't work very effectively, especially in the long-term. As the current health and fitness world is plagued with lose weight quick schemes and dramatic before and after's, the smoke and mirror lies can easily have you believing that this is what you need to be doing to re-shape and lose the weight.

That's why I wanted to write this chapter and walk you through how a small introduction of yin focused movement can fast-track your results. As for me, I have at least one day a week that I call my 'yinday.' It's a day where I read, meditate, spend undistracted time with family and friends, walk, stretch, surf, and whatever else will help me just chill out and stop being such an A-type personality.

Once a day, I want to be doing something that is yin focused. And this is where for over two years now, I've walked every morning. It's become a part of my morning routine that I love. The beauty of walking is that it's going to help you:

- De-stress.
- Aid your recovery from your other workouts.
- Help stabilize blood sugars.
- Burn more energy and fat.
- NOT have the risk of burning lean muscle tissue like sprints or interval training.
- Make you more productive.

Normally, a very confused face comes starring back at me when I tell people that I walk every day. For me, this is a part of my morning routine that gets me productive for the day to come and also comes along with a host of benefits.

This is where <u>balance</u> is so important. If I just wrote the above sections about MRT and Met Con trading and stopped there, you would be trying to fit as many high-intensity sessions in per week: On a fast-track to burning out and creating other issues with your body and health that can only slow or even stop your fat loss.

To be perfectly honest, the main reason I love to walk in the mornings is to give my brain space to think and have the time to be creative. As walking is shown to improve memory and brain performance as shown in this Stanford study (38).

I know you picked up this book because you wanted to get into amazing shape, and that's certainly going to happen. But I've got another agenda, and that is to give you great health and help you be the best person you can be. And that means the mental performance of your life is going to get a huge boost.

As a part of the programs, a very basic behavior focus goal is the number of steps you take each day. And this starts off with the target of having over 10,000 steps each day. With a short 20-minute walk and being conscious of how much you're moving this isn't a high number.

Going back to the balance of Yin and Yang, we go through periods of time in our lives when demands are greater, and the stress load is heavier. Stress can come from a range of factors, such as malnutrition, toxicity, relationship difficulties, financial struggles, work problems, pushing "all-nighters," taking stimulants (such as caffeine of 'fat burner' supplements), and more. We may turn to food for comfort in these times, and as I've previously covered, There are physiological changes that happen in our bodies.

Our adrenal glands are a part of the system that governs our stress response, and when they are overworked, the body can shift into an issue called 'adrenal imbalance' or 'adrenal fatigue.' That can then shift your body to store fat and calories, making it incredibly difficult to lose weight.

Here's where it gets interesting. Scientists have discovered that fat cells actually have special receptors for the stress hormone, cortisol, and there are more of these receptors in our abdominal fat cells than anywhere else in our bodies. In addition, scientists have shown that belly fat is actually an active tissue, acting as an endocrine organ that responds to the stress response by actually welcoming more fat to be deposited! This is an ongoing cycle, until we take steps to correct this adrenal imbalance.

How Can Adrenal Problems Lead to Weight Gain?

What's the reason behind this centralized adiposity?

According to author of Fat Chance, Dr. Robert Lustig, "belly fat breaks down into fatty acids faster, and has a direct line to the liver for burning." Basically, our body can get to the fat faster when we need it in times of physical emergency.

The single biggest contributing factor to adrenal fatigue (or an adrenal imbalance, as I like to call it) is stress. It sounds simple enough, but the reality is that stress comes in so many varieties and forms that it's impossible to avoid altogether. What we must do is identify the forms that we can best control in our lives, and work on making diet and lifestyle modifications to work on lowering the stress load on our systems. We can also work on finding better ways to help our bodies to manage the stressors that we do experience which we cannot eliminate.

Now honestly, I'm not going to dig deep into the huge problem that adrenal imbalance can be. That deserves its own book, and I will add to the resources section, Great Reads ones that I recommend on this topic from experts that I highly respect.

I wanted to bring up the relationship between adrenal imbalance and the stressors in life that can stop you from getting the health and body you want, because this is a serious problem I see frequently.

For years now, I've had both male and female clients come to me utterly fed up and frustrated. Having "tried all the diets" and training with personal trainers and even seen doctors, they have not been able to lose weight, or feel normal again.

A great example of this is Melanie. A late twenties personal trainer who has competed as a bikini model. When she came to me, she wanted to lose the 8-10 kilos that had been gained at a dramatic speed after stepping on stage as a bikini model. And unfortunately, this is a common theme with both male and female competitors, though I see it more often with females. This could just be that I have more female clients come to me in these situations, or another reason could be that I think females have a lower tolerance to stress, thyroid, and adrenal issues.

Melanie was back to eating close to her pre-competition diet in an effort to lose the excess weight, which was a low-calorie, low-carb, highly restrictive meal plan. Being a fitness model and having competed before, I know from a "how to make the diet work for me" situation that you have to only eat a very select amount of foods. I've certainly done it the wrong way before, and when eating such a small amount of foods, you have a restricted amount of nutritional value.

So onto the low calories, and carbs. Melanie also had a low nutrition density in her diet, which can lead to or flare up other problems from not having the nutrients, vitamins, minerals, and enzymes in her diet.

But, let's focus on just the training side of the equation to what got Melanie, and many others in her similar situation, to burn off the excess fat, and actually start feeling normal again by not dealing with a rollercoaster of mood and energy swings.

Starting with the lowering of overall total training volume. Her weight training workouts were effectively halved in time. With the introduction of MRT style workouts, we were able to produce a much greater fat-loss effect and not over train or over stress her body. Then it was substituting her interval training cardio with walking, and what suited her lifestyle was a 30-minute walk each afternoon.

She was already waking early for her work, so I didn't want her to be waking even earlier; as another big focus was making sure she improved the quality of her sleep and got over seven and a half hours of shut-eye each night. So morning walks weren't going to suit her schedule, which is perfectly fine. And the reason I wanted to highlight this is so that you don't get caught up with trying to follow the 'fasted cardio' crowd or any other specific tactic for fat loss. It's making it fit in with you, so that you can easily and happily follow it for the long-term success.

Then we introduced one (and soon after two, because she enjoyed it so much) #yindays. Where she did yoga and spent time laying down in the sun reading. There was no high-intensity training on these days.

The outcome was dramatic as she started burning off the body fat and enjoying much greater energy and wellbeing throughout the day. Literally turning into a new person, which I found out was the <u>real</u> Melanie, one who wasn't weighed down with restrictive diets or crazy high-training schedules.

I wanted to share Melanie's story with you because this is like many other success stories that have come about by being smarter, and not just going harder or trying to do more. And why you are going to be using #yinday and including walking, stretching, and meditation as a part of your transformation plan.

If you want to shrug this off and add more weight training sessions and intense cardio, I get it. I was exactly like that, but you have to realize that you can't keep banging your head against the wall, doing the same things and expecting a different result. I dare you to include and use the entire plans as I have designed for you, so you can watch your body, and feel the difference as you transform.

This is also why the outlined programs that I have for you, and especially in the free downloads section, are going to have already mapped out the steps you can take to easily maintain this balance. So you're accelerating your fat loss, improving your health, and easily fitting this into your lifestyle.

29

INNER GAME - GOAL SETTING AND WILLPOWER

Have you ever thought…

"Why does a smart person like myself struggle with something like losing weight?"

As the truth is, it's not a straightforward fix of just 'eating less and moving more.'

We have already covered how the power of the brain works with the body to determine if you are the healthy, fit, lean, strong, confident self that you say that you want to be. But this book, and the plans and programs to be successful need to include what I'm about to give you.

One of the biggest reasons why so many diets and weight loss programs haven't worked for you is because they fail to understand that one of the biggest building blocks of nutrition is your relationship with food.

The great Sufi poet, Rumi, once remarked: "The satiated man and the hungry man do not see the same thing when they look upon a loaf of bread." how each of us thinks about eating is so profoundly relative that if a group of us were looking at the same plate of food, no two people would see the same thing, or metabolize it the same way.

For example, let's look at a plate of chicken, salad, and bread. An athlete could look at this and see the protein and carbs as building blocks of performance and recovery. A woman wanting to lose weight could be scared of the bread, and want to pick at the chicken and salad. A vegan would not want to have the chicken. A farmer would be proud of the fresh produce that's gone from land to plate. A scientist could see a collection of chemicals.

And what the amazing and important part of you is that everyone is going to metabolize this meal differently, in accordance to their thoughts. In other words, what you think and feel about a food can be as important a determinant of its nutritional value and its effect on body weight as the actual nutrients themselves.

Now, you might possibly be thinking I've gone a little nuts to include this in the book. But stay with me for just a minute, and I'll show you how this works.

As I talked about in the Refuel Meals chapter, the parasympathetic and autonomic nervous system can be stimulated differently depending on how you view and feel about a food or meal you are eating. For example, let's talk about eating ice cream.

If you're feeling guilty about eating the ice cream or judging yourself for eating it, the hypothalamus will take this negative input and send signals down the sympathetic fibers of the autonomic nervous system. This action initiates inhibitory responses in the digestive organs, which means you'll be eating your ice cream but not fully metabolizing it. It may stay in your digestive system longer, which can diminish your population of healthy gut bacteria and increase the release of toxic by-products into the bloodstream. Furthermore, inhibitory signals in the nervous system can decrease your calorie-burning efficiency via increased insulin and cortisol, which would cause you to store more of your guilt-infused ice cream as body fat. So the thoughts you think about the food you eat instantly become reality in your body via the central nervous system.

This is why I don't want you to feel guilty or shame while eating. These judgments can be considered as stressors, and the brain will act to create its electrochemical equivalents in the body. You could eat the healthiest meal on the planet, but if you're thinking toxic thoughts, the digestion of your food goes down, and your fat storage metabolism can go up. Likewise, you could be eating a nutritionally challenged meal, but if your head and heart are in the right place, the nutritive power of your food will be increased.

And this is why I'm going to walk you through the placebo effect, and how it plays a big part of your nutrition and results.

You Are the Placebo

It took me a long time to first discover that there was a mind over metabolism power. And it then took some convincing for me to see the importance of this. We've covered how your body can metabolize foods and meal differently depending on how you look at it. And that our subconscious and identity that we create for ourselves helps us act or not act on certain things. It's now important to use the placebo effect to your advantage.

Marc David introduced me to this extraordinary example of the force the placebo effect plays.

In 1983, medical researchers were testing a new chemotherapy treatment. One group of cancer patients received the actual drug being tested while another group received a placebo – a fake harmless, inert chemical substance. As you may know, pharmaceutical companies are required by law to test all new drugs against a placebo to determine the true effectiveness, if any, of the product in question. In the course of this study, no one thought twice when 74 percent of the cancer patients receiving the real chemotherapy exhibited one of the more common side effects of this treatment: they lost their hair. Yet, quite remarkably, 31 percent of the patients on the placebo chemotherapy – an inert saltwater injection – also had an interesting side effect: they lost their hair too. Such is the power of expectation. The only reason that those placebo patients lost their hair is because they believed they would. Like many people, they associated chemotherapy with going bald.

If your hair can fall out from the thoughts you have. How important do you believe thinking "this chocolate tastes good, but it's really fattening, and I shouldn't be having it."

All I'm suggesting is that there is a power behind the thoughts and beliefs you have. And it would be wrong of me not to take this into account on how you, me, and everyone else transforms their body and health. This is a reason why I broke this book down to dispel the common myths, to show you what really matters when it comes to burning off the unwanted weight. As I've always found an educated client is an adherent client.

And this is also so that your beliefs and thoughts around what you need to be doing to look, feel, and function throughout each day can be aligned with what gets you those results. Can you now see that the potency of your expectations plays a role in what those results you get actually are?

Researchers have estimated that 35 to 45 percent of all prescription drugs may owe their effectiveness to placebo power, and that 67 percent of all over-the-counter medications, such as headache remedies, cough medicines, and appetite suppressants, are also placebo based. In some studies, the response to placebos is as high as 90 percent.

For me, the connection between placebo and food is strong. And for me to best coach and help you and my members to get the best results possible, it's my duty to use every tool in my arsenal to the best use at the right time. And this is what I want for you. Indeed, the placebo effect is built into the nutritional process. It's profoundly present on a day to day basis every time we eat. What we believe is alchemically translated into the body through nerve pathways, the endocrine system, neuropeptide circulation, the immune network, and the digestive tract.

This is so you can bring a happier and relaxed you to the table and each meal. Ultimately giving you the body and health you want, and enjoying the process.

Your Identity and Your Subconscious

I laughed, as it actually happened just last night.

Sitting down to dinner, a friend was reading through the menu.

His eyes locked onto something and kept coming back to it.

I could tell he was battling with what to choose, and that he really wanted this one dish.

Within a few minutes, he did just what I mentioned in the "Death of Cheat Meals."

"Screw it… I'll start on Monday."

As I nearly lost my coconut water through my nose with laughter. I had to talk him through the psychology of what was happening.

We can all justify something to ourselves so easily in the moment.

We can say to ourselves, "I've been training really hard this week, I deserve it." Or, "Why not, I've got to live a little."

Intellectually, that rationale makes complete sense. Suddenly, you have a perfectly legitimate reason to devour your favorite carb-loaded, sugary, fatty dish, and finish it off with a massive dessert.

Far from being an indulgence, that meal paves the way for hunger, cravings, weight loss resistance, and food intolerances. This is why when Monday rolls around, you can struggle to stick to the eating plan you've set yourself.

"I'll start Monday" falls into the self-sabotaging clichés that sound perfectly legitimate and yet highjack fat loss and optimal health. They stop you from becoming your very best self. And it gets deeper…

A fantastic book that I recommend to many is, "The Big Leap" by PhD Hendricks Gay. The book demonstrates how to eliminate the barriers to success by overcoming false fears and beliefs. And this is where you can be self-sabotaging yourself over and over, only standing in your own way to the results and achievements you want to attain.

This not only goes for your body and health. This pertains to your finances, relationships, and other areas of your life.

Often, we want something in our lives but behave in ways that conflict with us achieving our goals. The process of achieving that weight loss goal is a whole process, and at times, it can be an uncomfortable process. It's uncomfortable letting go of food and your beliefs that you may have firmly held for so long. You might feel resistant to finding new ways to treat yourself that do not involve the biscuit jar.

And this is where we can be our own worst enemies, and why I needed to include this chapter. It's my belief that without this, everything I have written previously is nearly worthless.

Self-sabotaging thoughts and behaviors are perpetuated by an inner critic we all possess, which psychologist and author, Robert Firestone, calls the "critical inner voice."

The critical inner voice doesn't represent a positive sense of self that you can trust in. Rather, it epitomizes a cruel "anti-self," a part inside us that is turned against us.

Our critical inner voice is formed from our early life experiences. Without realizing it, we tend to internalize attitudes that were directed toward us by parents or influential caretakers throughout our development. For example, if our parent saw us as lazy, we may grow up feeling useless or ineffective. We may then engage in self-sabotaging thoughts that tell us not to try, e.g. "Why bother? You'll never succeed anyway. You just don't have the energy to get anything done."

In a similar manner, children can internalize negative thoughts that their parents or early caretakers have toward themselves. If we grew up with a self-hating parent, who often viewed themselves as weak or a failure, we might grow up with similar self-sabotaging attitudes toward ourselves.

Personally, this is why, as a father of two beautiful daughters, I am working every day to be the best version of myself. And also, have my thoughts, actions, words, and behaviors be the best role model for them.

We can't change the past. Yet, as adults, we can identify the self-sabotaging thoughts that we've internalized and consciously choose to act against them. When we fall victim to our critical inner voice and listen to its directives, we often engage in self-limiting or self-sabotaging behaviors that hurt us in our daily lives. As author, Elizabeth Gilbert, put it, "You need to learn how to select your thoughts just the same way you select your clothes every day. This is a power you can cultivate. If you want to control things in your life so bad, work on the mind. That's the only thing you should be trying to control."

Why is it so common that people lose weight, and put it on again?

I think it's because the diet and weight loss plan they were trying to follow wasn't right for their body or for their lifestyle. However, I also think it goes deeper. There are several reasons why we lose weight and then regain it, along with a few extra pounds. Some people feel distinctly uncomfortable or awkward when they receive compliments or attention on their weight loss. Others can be anxious about the increased sense of personal power or confidence that weight loss will bring.

It's an identity shift that has to happen. So let me walk you through how I see this works:

Our identity determines our thoughts.

Our thoughts determine our actions.

Our actions determine our results.

Most people are totally focused on just gritting their teeth and using willpower to force themselves to take the right actions. But numerous cognitive neuroscientists have conducted studies that have revealed that only 5% of our cognitive activities (decisions, emotions, actions, behavior) are conscious, whereas the remaining 95% are generated in a non-conscious manner.

And this is where I believe the start is with self-love.

You either love being lean and vibrant with energy and a nourished body. Or you love to jump on the couch, eat pizza and ice cream, staying up late binge-watching a TV series.

You have to accept that your conscious choices are a result of what you truly love. And this is why combining the small, easy to use steps I walk you through in the My Body Diet create the habits and behaviors that doing the things that give you the body and health you want on autopilot.

You also need to accept that you can treat yourself. And you should take care of yourself. Abundance is not a mental thought, it's the action that you take that helps concrete in an abundant mindset. And I'm not talking about eating an abundant amount of ice cream. I'm talking about being able to have the body, the vibrant health, the loving relationships, the financial freedom, and the life that you really want deep down.

This is why cultivating a belief of gratitude is so powerful. As what you appreciate, appreciates. So next time you bite into a sweet, delicious, nutrient-rich strawberry that tingles your senses, be grateful that you have chosen to nourish yourself over choosing pancakes. As it's transformation on the inside that creates the transformation on the outside.

Personally, I find it astonishing that I just wrote the above. Not long ago, I would have scoffed if someone had said that to me about the psychology of self-sabotage, the placebo effect, why our identity, subconscious and self-love are intimate and important factors of life. But it's what I see now as true. And it's combing the science and anecdotal evidence of nutrition, training, supplements, and lifestyle factors, along with the deep inner work that truly creates a plan that gives you the results you really want.

It was when I first learned about the observer effect that my beliefs and how I transformed myself and my clients all changed.

One of the premises of quantum theory, which has long

fascinated philosophers and physicists alike, states that by the very act of watching, the observer affects the observed reality. According to a 2002 poll of Physics World readers, the "most beautiful experiment" in physics is one that simply and elegantly demonstrates how observation affects quantum systems. The experiment revealed that the greater the amount of "watching," the greater the observer's influence on what actually takes place.

Don't worry, I'm not going to delve into the world of quantum physics right now. I just want you to understand that if you've been following the traditional diet and weight loss advice and it hasn't worked for you, It's not your fault.

And this is why I've found it so amazing that dozens of interviews with the world's top coaches and experts have always turned to the mental side for when it comes to truly being able to transform and get results.

One such powerful interview was with Ben Coomber. As within just a few minutes of us starting our interview, our conversation was on what the usual mental blocks are. And as Ben puts it, "perhaps it's the way you think, the way you are wired, your upbringing, and just how you feel about yourself. Either way, the way you think and act might be holding you back." And it's by including the plan, program, advice, help, and information that gives you the tools and tactics to be able to skipper mental road blocks.

Does This Sound Familiar..?

With over 10 years of coaching people to transform their body, there has been a common thread that I hear when a client first comes to me.

It often goes like this:

Client: "I want to finally be able to lose this weight. I've tried everything."

Me: "Great, tell me what you're currently doing to lose the weight?"

Client: "Well, I usually have to wake up at 6am so I can go for a run and be back in time to get everything ready for the kids to go to school. Then, I'm out the door, off to work. I try to eat healthy during the day, but work is so busy."

Me: "What do you usually eat during work?"

Client: "It's normally a coffee and a protein bar around midmorning if I feel like I'm losing my energy. I try to have a salad at lunch, but it's usually a sandwich I've had to pick up that I eat at the computer, or trying to eat healthy when taking clients out for lunches."

Me: "How does the rest of the day look?"

Client: "I'll get home famished, and try to fit a workout in. But then it's getting dinner ready which is usually a meat, vegetables, or a pasta with a wine to help me relax and unwind. But I always crave chocolate or something sweet after dinner."

And the conversation continues… Which is a common theme of trying to do so many different things, and trying to stick to guidelines of nutrition and exercise that just don't fit with a lifestyle. It's like trying to get a square peg through a round hole.

This is why I want you to focus on only what is essential, and we have set up the steps for you to follow. As things get easier by first subtracting, take away the number of things you are trying to do, and 'rules' you have to stick to.

What is essential - it gets easier by subtracting.

The importance of habits, and why I'll show you how to set the right ones up

You Are Your Habits

What if I told you that you could lose weight while continuing to eat all your favorite foods?

You'd call me crazy, but I'd tell you it's the easier way. Think about your last low-carb diet; how long did it take until you caved and just ordered a pizza? I'd bet it was much sooner than you'd like to admit.

You see, the reason dropping those first few pounds is so difficult is because the majority of weight loss strategies begin by eliminating foods from your diet. While that certainly makes sense, stacking up major diet change on top of major diet change is not only overwhelming, it can also make you feel deprived and disheartened. As a result, you might lose weight initially, but it can just as easily come right back.

Have you ever noticed how you can get a really strong urge to eat something that you know you are trying limit? And the urge and craving just get stronger and stronger?

One piece of research at Cornell found how strong food and screen cravings can affect our behavior when he noticed how Cinnabon stores were located in shopping malls. Most food stores in shopping malls are all next to each other in a food court. However,

Cinnabon intentionally located away from all other food stores so they could have the smell of cinnamon scrolls waft down the isles so that shoppers will subconsciously start craving a roll. So, by the time the shopper walks around the corner and gets up to the store, the craving has grown and is consuming the thoughts of the shopper.

Wolfram Schultz, a professor of neuroscience at the University of Cambridge said, "There is nothing programmed into our brains that makes us see a box of doughnuts and automatically want a sugary treat… But once our brain learns that a doughnut box contains yummy sugar and other carbohydrates, it will start anticipating the sugar high. Our brains will push us toward the box. Then, if we don't eat the doughnut, we'll feel disappointed."

You can see through the work of Schultz and what has emerged with neuroscience and the understanding of habits and how our brains work, that it can be easy to be wired for eating the wrong foods, and struggling with starting new habits that get you exercising, eating the right foods, and getting to bed on time, etc. However, these cravings don't have complete authority over us. As I'll walk you through what it is you can do, and why we've designed the My Body Diet to build the mechanisms in place for you to ignore the temptations and have the right habits in place that make it automatic for you losing weight and keeping it off.

During their extensive studies of the underpinnings of habit in the 1990s, researchers at the Massachusetts Institute of Technology discovered a simple neurological loop at the core of every habit.

The process within our brains is a three-step loop. First, there is a cue, a trigger that tells your brain to go into automatic mode and which habit to use. Then there is a routine, which can be physical or mental or emotional. Finally, there is a reward, which helps your brain figure out that this particular loop is worth remembering for the future. And then, the fourth factor added, being a craving is how you can set yourself up for success, or be stuck in a spiral of yo-yo dieting. I learned this from the brilliant work of Charles Duhigg, who has written The Power of Habits, and more recently, Smarter Faster Better. Both books I recommend.

We now know why habits emerge, how they change, and the science behind the mechanics. We know how to break them into parts and rebuild them to our specifications. We understand how to make people eat less, exercise more, and live healthier lives.

"We've done experiments where we trained rats to run down a maze until it was a habit, and then we extinguished the habit by changing the placement of the reward" Ann Gabryiel, a scientist at MIT said. "Then one day, we'll put the reward in the old place, and put in the rat, by golly, the old habit will re-emerge right away. Habits never really disappear. They're encoded into the structures of our brain, and that's a huge advantage for us, because it would be awful if we had to relearn how to drive after every vacation. The problem is that your brain can't tell the difference between bad and good habits, and so if you have a bad one, it's always lurking there, waiting for the right cues."

Learning from Ann Gabriel, we can see this is why so many people struggle with trying to lose weight. Creating a habit to go out and exercise rather than sitting on the couch when you get home, for example. Those patterns always remain the same inside our heads. And this is why we can now use simple methods knowing the science so that we can create new neurological routines that overpower those behaviors.

To understand your own habits, you need to identify the components of your loops. Once you have diagnosed the habit loop of a particular behavior, you can look for ways to supplant old vices with new routines.

A great example is one that Charles gives of himself. "Let's say you have a bad habit, like I did when I started researching this book, of going to the cafeteria and buying a chocolate chip cookie every afternoon. Let's say this habit has caused you to gain a few pounds. In fact, let's say this habit has caused you to gain exactly 8 pounds, and that your wife has made a few pointed comments. You've tried to force yourself to stop – you even went so far as to put a post-it on your computer that reads "NO MORE COOKIES".

But every afternoon you manage to ignore that note, get up, wander toward the cafeteria, buy a cookie and, while chatting with colleagues around the cash register, eat it. It feels good, and then it feels bad. Tomorrow, you promise yourself, you'll muster the willpower to resist. Tomorrow will be different.

But tomorrow, the habit takes hold again."

How do you start diagnosing and then changing this behavior? By figuring out the habit loop. And the first step is to identify the routine. In this cookie scenario – as with most habits – the routine is the most obvious aspect: it's the behavior you want to change. Your routine is that you get up from your desk in the afternoon, walk to the cafeteria, buy a chocolate chip cookie and eat it while chatting with friends.

This is why we start with a 3-day food log. It's a truthful, objective look into what you're currently feeding yourself right now. Not only has it been shown that you're going to make better and healthier decisions by just doing this alone, you're also going to be able to find out what habits you're in.

When you can see that you're always going for the chocolate after dinner, or that your mid-morning snack is a carb-rich energy pick me up, it's easy to look for the cue that is starting your habit. This is why, by combining the physiological methods, such as eating good amounts of fats, fiber, and protein, along with setting up new habits, has you killing off cravings and set you up for success without the struggles.

Once I learned this, I spent months continually working on and perfecting what steps I can take someone through so that they are able to lose weight quickly to begin with, and so that they keep their motivation and not have to struggle with a lack results. But importantly, these steps set you up with habits and routines that fit into your life, so that you get into the body shape you want and stay in shape, never having to constantly battle with yo-yo or deprivation dieting.

This is why I also have the important Downloads and Coaching section that you can sign up for free by having this book. You'll be matched with the best meal plan and workout guide, along with the coaching sessions I've personally recorded; to walk you through the process of setting you up with the right habits. Go to http://cravingthetruth.com/bookbonus to get free access.

There are three habits that we look at setting up, working on one at a time.

1. Decide on what your reward is (without food).

In 2002, researchers at New Mexico State University studied 266 individuals, most of whom worked out at least three times a week. What they found was that they continued to exercise because of a specific reward they started to crave. In one group, 92% of people said that they habitually exercise because it made them "feel good." They grew to expect and crave the endorphins and other neurochemicals a workout gave them. In another group, 67% of people said that working out was a sense of "accomplishment." They had come to crave a regular sense of triumph from self-reward, which was enough to make a physical activity into a habit.

And this is why, in the coaching guide, we want to set you up with a cue, a reward and craving for that. And by first deciding on what your reward is, you can break old habits and start the process of forming new ones. And this is why the second habit you can start is…

2. Eliminate distractions while eating.

It is too easy in this busy, social media filled world to be sitting down watching something online, scrolling through social media, or replying back to messages and emails. This ties back into what we learned from Marc David and the psychology of eating, and how we need to have a connection of what we are actually putting into our mouths and bodies.

By first becoming conscious of what you're eating, you're going to be able to make smarter decisions in what foods you're choosing, and also, what habits are currently in place that you can overpower with new behaviors. Which again, works directly into the next habit…

3. Clean out your pantry and fridge.

If you're in the habit of going into the pantry and getting chocolate after dinner, then one way to break the habit is not have the food in the house to start with. I highly recommend that you go through your pantry and fridge and clean out all the foods that you know could be trigger foods, or temptations, or foods you don't want to be eating. And then go and donate those foods, and get them out of your home.

Now, my wife, Lauren, loves to eat chocolate. But she and I are very different in some ways. I'm more of an "all or nothing" person. Lauren, on the other hand, can have one or two squares of dark chocolate after dinner and be totally satisfied, but also many nights just happily saying no to it. I think on a psychological side, she has a much healthier stance. Me on the other hand, having battled with binge eating before, I know that I need to be smart about not falling into old habits.

So, therefore, after dinner, the first thing I do is make myself a cup of tea. Either a peppermint or ginger tea with turmeric. This simply replaced the routine of finishing dinner, and then going on the couch and watching TV while eating chocolate. Then we made another change as we became conscious about setting up what we did to best give us what we want. Instead of plugging into Netflix or a TV series, we replaced it with reading or going onto our balcony to just kick back, relax, and talk.

Not only am I not eating chocolate or having any cravings for it, I'm connecting with quality time with my wife. And this is where this book is about so much more than losing weight. In all honesty, I know that our egos are strong and being able to lose weight to look better is a strong driving factor, but life is more than just what body fat you eat. And this is why I want to put your health first, so you can thrive and be the best version of you.

Outcome Versus Behavior Focused.

One of the ingredients that makes up the 'secret sauce' for success with transforming bodies comes down to a simple mind switch that I learned from Dr. John Berardi.

It was one of the most important coaching changes I made, and it felt like every single client and member that I used this hack with had the ability to relax, enjoy life, and get faster results. And simply it is this…

Most people are focused on how much weight they want to be losing overall, or per week.

They think "I've got to lose 2 pounds every week." Or -

"I want to get down to 60kg."

The simple problem with this is that you are constantly focusing on the end goal. But that's not what gets you there. And the big problem is that how your body responds, is not what is in your control. What you are able to control are your actions.

The actions and behaviors you take, as in the small steps, build-up into getting you where you want to go.

So rather than constantly thinking of the outcome being the

end goal you want to accomplish, focus on what are the key actions or behaviors that you need to be doing per day that get you to your end goal.

If you're focusing on "I will follow my meal plan today," or "I will make my workout today," these behaviors are the actions that are needed to get you to your end goal, and is what allows you to stop stressing over the gap between where you are right now, and the end goal that might seem so far away.

This simple switch of mastering the behavior goals consistently over time is what will get you the results you want, and also bring you peace, as you are focusing on something that actually is in your control.

Now that we have covered the Inner Game and The Power of Habits, it's now time for us to go into the two important lifestyle factors.

What It All Starts With

> "You must own everything in your world. There is no one else to blame"
>
> – Jocko Willink

Victor Frankl shows you how even in the most awful of situations a human being can be put in, there is still the one, underlying principle that you and I need to live by.

His book, 'Mans Search For Meaning,' he chronicles his experiences as a concentration camp inmate, which led him to discover the importance of finding meaning in all forms of existence, even the most brutal ones, and thus, a reason to continue living. And what does this have to do with you transforming your body and health…

Even when all your possessions are taken from you, when you have lost love, when living in absolute destitute, it is still the power that we hold in ourselves to perceive and make what we want with what happens with the outside world.

I had to first read the book twice, from front to back. As the first time I read it, I knew I wasn't grasping everything I had to. I knew that my own ego was playing victim. And I could play victim, and lie to myself saying that there are always reasons outside of my control that determine what happens in my life.

If could be:

"I have bad genetics that makes it so easy for me gain weight."

"I just can't lose the weight no matter what I do."

"My husband doesn't want to make lifestyle and food changes that I want to make, and it makes it too hard for me."

Telling ourselves those lies gives our ego the winning edge. But it disempowers us. And will never allow us to truly break free of the problems and live the lives that we really want.

This is exactly why I named My Body Blends, what it is. It's you talking to yourself. It's bringing together all the factors of food, movement, lifestyle, supplementation and blending it into the mix that is right for YOU.

Just last week, I wrote a post quoting Jesse Elder, and it's a perfect fit for you here.

"You are operating perfectly. You are operating perfectly to create in your own experience everything that you are currently getting." - Jesse Elder

This empowers to realize that the answer lies within yourself and what you are doing.

The starting conversation that made this 'click' for me was with Mark Buckley. The founder of FMA Strength Institute, but also a man I highly respect who is very well rounded in his approach to not only training, but life. He was the first person who opened up the world of 'self-parenting.'

The idea of **self-parenting** is that a person's "mind" is created in the form of a conversation between two voices generated by the two parts of the cerebral hemisphere. One is the "inner parent" represented by the left brain with the other voice being the "inner child "represented by the right brain. The manner and quality by which these "inner conversations" take place between the two voices are most accurately described as self-parenting. The inner parent is parenting the inner child within the inner conversations.

As this puts the power into your hands. It's by ensuring you are equipped with the right information, that you can now take this and put it into action. Only then, does this information turn into wisdom by it being combined with experience.

Personally I have learnt a lot from Ben Pakulski. A former elite level bodybuilder, that is now helping men across the world build the bodies that they want, but also build the lives that they want. It's one of Ben's strengths to understand and coach people to have a much greater quality of training. Through employing the best methods and strategies in training program design and execution. His results with himself and his users are world class.

But this also goes into the importance of your mental focus not just inside your workouts, but through everyday life. Much of this book have been influenced by what I have learnt from Ben and been able to then prove with myself and members.

I cannot, and no one can, give you the perfect diet or weight loss program. And it's by using the principles as a foundation, and knowledge that I give you here, where I want you to take ownership of your own results. And you can go out and make the smart choices to become who you want to be.

And it's having this that I now want to continue to give you the arsenal of tools to do just that.

30
LIFESTYLE

Here's a quick question for you;

What is the #1 reason most people fail to lose weight and keep it off?

In my experience, the answer is simple.

As when I was gathering all the research material for writing this book, I came across Dr. Mark Hyman, saying that, "The average person gains 11 pounds for every diet they go on."

The cruel fact is that traditional dieting is making it harder and harder for you to lose weight. The key to losing weight and keeping it off are two simple things. First, automatically reduce your appetite, not by white knuckling it and starving yourself, but fixing the out of whack hormones and brain chemistry that drive hunger and overeating.

The second is to automatically increase your metabolism so you burn more calories all day long. Unfortunately, most diets do the opposite – increase hunger and slow metabolism.

Here's the deal…

I've received thousands of emails from people that are training hard and eating "healthy."

And they are battling on a day by day basis as to why it's so hard to stick to the plan, and to finally lose the weight.

You can be doing everything right with your diet and training. But if you are skating through each day with a lack of sleep and trying to juggle an overload of stress, you're sabotaging yourself. Your body and brain are going to fight back against you.

And this is why I'm going to show you the quick and effective hacks, so that you can wake up each day beaming with energy, have the mental performance to be the best version of yourself, and have your body burning body fat faster than ever before.

Sleep

Do you know someone (and this could be you) that struggles to maintain mental focus? Has trouble controlling their hunger, always craving sweets, and despite their biggest efforts in the gym, they don't seem to achieve the same results as someone else following the same program?

The problem might seem obvious at first. After all, they always stray from their diet more than others. And if exercise "isn't working," it probably means they just don't really know how to train.

Maybe it's genetics. Maybe they're lazy or lack willpower. Or maybe, diet or exercise isn't the real problem.

It could be that the missing link for your weight loss success is… sleep.

Sleep deprivation causes hormone imbalance (leptin, Ghrelin, cortisol, you name it). These out of balance hormones wreak havoc with appetite and metabolism. The result? When you are low on sleep, you're more inclined consume extra calories, and you're less able to burn off the calories and fat you consume.

In fact, one study, presented at the Endocrine Society national meeting, suggests that getting just 30 fewer minutes sleep than you should per weekday can increase your risk of obesity and diabetes (96).

When you sleep less, you take in more calories. This can happen for several reasons related to your hormones. Changes in your glucose metabolism brought on by sleep deprivation will cause your body to hoard the calories you consume, storing them as fat rather than burning them for energy. Also, low sleep levels cause your body to produce more of the stress hormone, cortisol, which in turn, spurs your appetite.

The problems with sleep deprivation and sleep loss are:
- It reduces your insulin sensitivity (101). Your actual metabolic capacity to handle eating carbohydrates, that is to use them for energy instead of storing them as fat, gets harder. A reduction in insulin sensitivity means that you're more likely to store food as fat (and then still be hungry afterward).
- It changes the composition of your gut flora (102). We've

already covered the importance of your gut health, and being sure that your micro biome is populated with good bacteria that promotes health and weight loss.
- It also increases inflammation. In this study (103), for example, either sleeping 5 hours a night or sleeping at the wrong time (the shift work pattern), increased markers of inflammation. And this study (104) makes it even clearer: "sleep deficient humans…exhibit a proinflammatory component; therefore, sleep loss is considered as a risk factor for developing cardiovascular, metabolic, and neurodegenerative diseases (e.g., diabetes, Alzheimer's disease, and multiple sclerosis)."

Study after study has shown that if they're allowed to choose their own diet, sleep-deprived subjects will eat more food, especially more junk (99,100).

Research indicates that a body deprived of sleep burns calories less effectively than a well-rested one (97).

Michael Breus, PhD, a sleep specialist and author of The Sleep Doctor's Diet Plan: Lose Weight Through Better Sleep. Says "The more sleep deprived you are, the higher your levels of the stress hormone cortisol, which increases your appetite."

"When you're stressed, your body tries to produce serotonin to calm you down. The easiest way to do that is by eating high-fat, high-carb foods that produce a neurochemical reaction," Breus says.

A lack of sleep also hinders your body's ability to process carbohydrates. "When you're sleep deprived, the mitochondria in your cells that digest fuel start to shut down. Sugar remains in your blood, and you end up with high blood sugar," says Breus. Losing out on sleep can make fat cells 30 percent less able to deal with insulin, according to a study in Annals of Internal Medicine (98).

One reason you might pack on pounds when you're sleep deprived is because your body goes into survival mode. Sleeplessness can fool your body into thinking you're in danger. "Your metabolism slows because your body is trying to maintain its resources, and it also wants more fuel," says Breus. "I would argue that sleep is probably the most important thing a person can do if they're ready to start a diet and lose weight."

Luckily, there are easy ways to make sure sleep never gets in between you and your goal weight again. First, figure out your bedtime. Count seven and a half hours before the time you need to wake up, says Breus. That's your "lights out" time, which should ensure you're getting enough sleep to make your body wake itself up at the proper time (maybe even before an alarm goes off).

Janet K. Kennedy, PhD, clinical psychologist and founder of NYC Sleep Doctor, also says to keep your bed time and wake up time consistent. "Doing that and getting out of bed at the same time sets your body's clock so you'll be tired around the same time every night," she says.

Now there are easy solutions that can have a big impact, not only in the number of hours you sleep, but also the in the quality of your sleep. We can initially break it down into two steps that have proven time and again to be a simple fix that can not only help you lose weight, but feel and function better each day.

The Wind Down Routine:

Imagine this...

Instead of waking up and feeling groggy, and having the strong urge to just hit the snooze button and pull the warm and comfy sheets back over. Then going through the grind of starting your day, yet you're still half asleep and zombie-like trying to make yourself a coffee in a desperate attempt to slap yourself awake to get going with your day...

You woke up before your alarm even went off.

You woke up like a light. With your brain switched on and clear. You kick your legs out of bed and have simple clarity and the energy to thrive through the day.

But why isn't this happening now? Why is the groggy, slow, snooze button temptation the usual start to the day, rather than the switched on, go make the most of the day?

The biggest problem we face is our modern lifestyles are being constantly stimulated.

Social media companies spend millions on designing their platforms to addict us to keep checking our phones for updates. The ease of which you can switch on Netflix, and get hooked on an entire TV series, so not only are you binge-watching episode after episode, but your brain is super stimulated after watching.

Your brain isn't having the time or environment to wind down properly and switch off, which prepares you for an awesome night's sleep.

This is why we use the Wind Down Routine as our step one to making your sleep into a supercharger for each day to come.

Simply, you're going to start 30 minutes before you usually go to bed. You're still going to go to bed at the same time as you do now, as we are going to focus on getting better quality sleep first, then we can look at quantity in a new and improved way with step 2.

#1: Turn Off Your Electronics.

Your sleep is regulated by an "internal clock" that is also tied in with your melatonin.

And your body uses light as its main way to regulate your melatonin production. As our modern lives have electronics and screens everywhere, it's easy for us to fall out of sync from the day's rise and fall of the sun.

Scrolling through Facebook, finishing off emails, or even watching Netflix at night can all be exposing you to the blue light that has been shown to suppress melatonin and affect sleep (199).

Now abolishing all technology for when the sun goes down would be the optimal thing to do, but I don't feel that it's realistic. So the next best thing we can do is to turn off electronics 30 minutes before bed.

In all-time brilliant timing, I was walking out of an event in Austin, Texas, and I walked straight into James Swannick (who I've wanted to interview and deep dive into the subject of limiting 'blue light' before bed). James is the creator of Swannick Sleep, and the blue-blocking sunglasses that can limit your exposure to blue light.

Research has found that exposure to **blue light** suppresses the production of melatonin more than any other type of **light**. It is believed that the shorter wavelengths in **blue light** are what causes the body to produce less melatonin.

> "In terms of light and our brains, there is a spectrum of wavelengths that impacts the human circadian system," said David Earnest, a professor and circadian rhythms expert at the Texas A&M Health Science Center College of Medicine. "Blue light is the most sensitive side of the spectrum."

A study by the University of Toronto (219) found that during night shifts, those who wore glasses that blocked blue light wavelengths produced more melatonin than those who didn't. Other studies (220) have found that blue wavelengths suppress delta brainwaves, which induce sleep and boost alpha wavelengths, which create alertness.

> Another way to limit the amount of blue light you are exposed to toward the end of the day is to wear a pair of "blue blocking" sunglasses. My favorite are the Swannies from Swannick Sleep, as they actually look good and are high quality. By wearing a pair of these glasses, you can improve the quality of your sleep by filtering out harmful artificial blue light from electronic devices that shut down your body's natural melatonin production and disrupt your sleep.

Now this is the starting base, we can extend your Wind Down Routine to an hour and beyond. But when kicking this off, I've found most clients find it easiest to start with 30 minutes.

Also, if you do need to work from a computer late at night (sometimes I've got interviews or just last-minute deadlines that need to be hit), download a software called Flux (www.justgetflux.com). This takes the Blue Light out of the screen, and will help to reduce stimulation before going to bed.

#2: Chill Out.

Now that we've turned off your smartphones, tablets, TV's, and computers, we've got a 30-minute or longer window for you to chill out.

Personally, in the last month, my wife and I have been fine-tuning our own Wind-Down Routine. Our two daughters are tucked up and in bed by 7pm. And rather than jumping on the couch and watching TV, we have no more TV in our home and have either candles or a Himalayan Rock Salt Lamp in our lounge room. This has been accompanied with Jambo Superfoods CBD oil and a Foursigmatic Mushroom hot cocoa drink.

To figure out if this is actually working for me or now, I'm tracking my sleep very closely by using an Oura Ring. This is showing my how well I'm recovering each day, my Heart Rate Variability, and a deep breakdown of my sleep quality. And with about 4-weeks of me following this routine most nights, I'm seeing a big improvement in my recovery and how I am waking up ready to take on another day.

But to really make sure we can have great sleep and recovery, we need our bedroom set up properly... Which start with 3 simple steps.

#3: Dark, Quiet and Cool.

Simple, your bedroom should be pitch black, with no noise coming in and cool.

As we travel 3-4 months of each year, we are in and out of Air BnBs and it's not exactly ideal to be lugging around blackout blinds with us all over the world. If you can't stop outside light coming into your bedroom, then a sleeping mask can be a great hack.

This also goes for noise, if you live on a busy street or have outside noise coming in, then a pair of ear plugs will be a great addition and very cheap.

Finally, it's about staying cool.

For me, I can "run hot" and find that I'll be sleeping on top of the covers whilst my wife is two layers under trying to stay warm. Many resources recommend that 15-17 degrees Celsius or 60-67 degrees Fahrenheit is best.

When we are living in Bali, this means I have air-conditioning and a small fan in the room.

Is that optimal with the added elasticity in the room?

NO. But I believe it's better for me to sleep in a cool room so I'm not uncomfortable, and that I can get deep, restful sleep.

Step 2: The Power of Your Chronotype.

Honestly…

I could not believe the difference.

I had prided myself on being an early riser. For nearly 10 years as a personal trainer, I was waking up at 4:30am to get myself ready and in the gym for my 6am client. Then, for the past 2 years, I was working from home. Yet I kept up the early rising mentality. I was usually getting up at 5am so that I could get as much work as possible done. The "hustler" mentality was the driving force for me.

Then I listened to Dr. Michael Breus, who wrote, The Power Of When: Discover Your Chronotype. And I made the changes that day to how I now structure my days, and when I go to sleep and wake up.

Most advice concentrates on <u>what</u> to do, or <u>how</u> to do it, and ignores the <u>when</u> of success. But exciting new research proves there is a right time to do just about everything based on our biology and hormones. As Dr. Michael Breus proves in THE POWER OF WHEN, working with your body's inner clock for maximum health, happiness, and productivity is easy, exciting, and fun.

Every person has a master biological clock ticking away inside their brain, and dozens of smaller biological clocks throughout his or her body.

But, unlike a normal clock, not every person's biological clock keeps the same time or even the same pace. If you've ever heard someone say, "I'm not a morning person," well there's a reason for that. Some people are meant to be more productive in the morning than at night, and vice versa.

Believe it or not – your body has been programmed to function much better at certain times of the day than others. Based on general morningness and eveningness preferences, different people fall into different classifications, called "Chronotypes."

This is where I recommend the book, The Power Of When, but also highly recommend you go The Power Of When quiz, where you'll be able to discover which chronotype you are. You will get the answers given to you as to when you're going to want to go to bed and wake up.

As for me, my chronotype is a 'bear.' I wake up and go down with the sun. I'm better at training intensely later in the day, and have my best creativity time a few hours after waking with a small surge late afternoon. So the first thing I did after discovering this was change my bedtime to 9:30pm and waking up at 6am for when the sun was rising.

It made a huge difference, and now I stick to this routine as much as possible. The only times it wavers is if I'm traveling or we are going out for dinner and spending time with friends. Though I always still wake up at the same time and won't sleep in, preferring to get up at the same time to keep my biological clock the same, and taking a quick nap during the day if needed.

This first starts with you needing to decide when are you going to bed and waking up, starting with a seven and a half-hour window. You can also choose if you want a little more or less quantity of sleep, though this seems to be the best starting number as it coincides with our sleep cycles. Then give yourself a 2-week experiment. You're going to stick to this sleeping and waking up time. Then you can look back and see how you feel to then make any changes that you want.

I have included the direct link in the Free and Bonus section that you can get access to by having this book.

The end of this chapter finishes with five simple steps, and the last one is where I will walk you through three super simple steps to hi-jack your sleep and improve its quality.

Stress

Have you ever been lying in bed and your brain is still running at a hundred miles an hour? You've had a busy day, and you feel depleted from the day's stress, choices, and multiple responsibilities that you're balancing. Now that it's finally time for you to rest… you can't.

This is what we call "tired but wired." And it's tied into how your body's stress hormones such as cortisol, epinephrine, and norephedrine can help you burn off the unwanted weight, or make it harder for you to lose your belly fat.

On one side, we have 'gurus' and weight loss pill pushers telling you that by simply 'blocking cortisol' (with whatever they're selling), you're going to be able to acerbate your weight loss.

But on the other side, we can actually use the 'fight or flight' response to our advantage to enhance the fat burning process.

Cortisol, like every other hormone in the body, has a specific purpose, which includes regulating the energy levels of the body. It does this by moving energy from fat stores to tissues that need it and, when the body is under stress, by providing protein for conversion into energy.

Cortisol actually induces lipolysis (the breakdown of fat into usable energy, known as free fatty acids) and oxidation (the burning of those fatty molecules). **Acute cortisol spikes help with fat loss, which is part of the fat burning power of exercise.**

However, while cortisol increases whole-body lipolysis, it tends to spare abdominal fat (106). This starts to explain the chronically elevated cortisol levels that can be linked with abdominal obesity (107).

So it's not that we want to kill off cortisol. We want to be able to use it to our advantage, and not have high levels that persist for too long.

And this is where I want to first show you how to balance your elevated cortisol levels, as a typical busy, modern lifestyle that we live today can easily push our stress hormones out of balance.

Dr. Robert Sapolsky is a Professor of Neurology at Stanford University, and he wrote a book I highly recommend called, Why Zebras Don't Get Ulcers.

"Stress is anything in the external world that knocks you out of homeostatic balance," Sapolsky said. "Let's say you're a zebra, and a lion has leaped out, ripped your stomach out. . . this counts as being out of homeostatic balance."

For a zebra, though, stress has an extremely short if potentially deadly span; it was "three minutes of screaming terror," after which, the animal was either dead or once again roaming the Savannah and feeling safe. Human beings, on the other hand, have an "anticipatory stress response" that spins easily out of control, like a car losing traction on an icy slope.

"If you think you're about to be knocked out of homeostatic

balance and really aren't, and this happens on a regular basis, then you're being anxious. . . paranoid. . . profoundly human," Sapolsky said. The point is that humans, unlike primates, "can get stressed simply with thought, turning on the same stress response as does the zebra." And when that stress response is turned on chronically, "We get sick."

"The fact is," he said, "that some of us are fabulous at coping, and I want to spend to last few minutes looking at why some of our psyches deal with stress better than others."

He also mentioned one that was essential in dealing with stress: "having a shoulder to cry on." "The biggest predictor of mortality across the board for all infectious disease is the degree of social isolation versus social affiliation. People who live alone don't have someone to remind them to take their medicine every day and don't have healthy dinners. Social isolation, then, is a major health-risk factor."

This is one major reason why I put such a focus on creating the best environment for everyone with the My Body Blends community. The free group, where you not only get access to the guides, programs, and episodes, but joining the like-minded people just like you that create the support network you can't get anywhere else.

But before we dive into the steps you can take to deal with stress, feel better each day, and enhance your fat loss, let's…

Find a better way to deal with your stress.

There's a reason why many people eat as a way to cope with stress. Stress causes certain regions of the brain to release chemicals (specifically, opiates and neuropeptide-Y). These chemicals can trigger mechanisms that are similar to the cravings you get from fat and sugar. In other words, when you get stressed, your brain feels the addictive call of fat and sugar, and you're pulled back to junk food.

We all have stressful situations that arise in our lives. Learning to deal with stress in a different way can help you overcome the addictive pull of junk food. This could include simple breathing techniques or a short guided meditation. Or something more physical, such as exercise or making art.

The problem starts when cortisol levels stay high over a prolonged period of time, they can increase insulin resistance and hyperinsulinemia (108). Consistently high blood glucose levels along with insulin suppression lead to cells that are starved of glucose. But those cells are crying out for energy, and one way to regulate this is to send hunger signals to the brain. This can lead to overeating. And, of course, unused glucose, along with overeating, is eventually going to lead to fat gain.

But the problem continues to spiral and get worse.

The relationship between stress and overeating has been thoroughly researched. Louisiana State University conducted a literature review, and found that as stress hormones like cortisol increase, so do ghrelin levels (ghrelin is the hormone that stimulates appetite). This hunger drives us to eat more and sometimes even to binge (109).

On top of becoming hungrier, it has also been shown that your stress can have you preferring "comfort foods" (110). The high-fat, high carb, high in calorie foods that can just lead to further overeating.

This Is How We Accelerate Your Fat Loss

When hormones levels are in balance, cortisol has many positive effects and helps you burn fat. For example, when you start working out, you can have a cascade of hormonal changes. Such as cortisol, catecholamines, and Growth Hormone being elevated. And this is done so that your body can free fat from its stores and can "burn fat" for energy. Also, your insulin levels will be lowered, further creating a better fat burning environment, because when cortisol is higher and insulin is lower, a fat burning enzyme called hormone sensitive lipase (HSL) gets elevated, and your fat storing enzyme lipoprotein lipase (LPL) is lowered.

This is one reason why I designed the workouts as the way they are to help further this fat burning process, and also, why the meal plan is structured to enable the best use of this fat burning hormone environment. For example, all these positive effects can be disrupted if you have a higher carb meal or drink too soon before training.

31

5 STEPS TO BALANCING STRESS, ACCELERATING YOUR FAT LOSS AND FEELING LIKE "YOU" AGAIN

Start with the My Body Diet.
We start with two things. Focusing on what goes in your mouth and what goes out your mouth.

Foundation of nutrient-dense foods that will help lower inflammation and take the stress out of all the questions we can have when it comes to food. Such as "what, when, and how much do I eat?"

Mindfulness Practice - 2min of breathing to 20min of meditation

I mentioned in the last point that we need to be conscious of what comes "out of our mouths." I'm a strong believer in the power of words, and how positive or negative is what you say, and who you surround yourself with. This is why the step of starting a Mindfulness Practice is so powerful.

By first working on yourself and even starting with just 2 minutes that can be purely focused on your breath (Vipassana meditation) or even using an app such as Stress Doctor.

Then if you want, you can start or build into meditation. Personally, I meditate for 20 minutes every morning. Granted, I will miss a few here or there depending on what's going on, but I've built the habit of at least getting a breathing and mindfulness session in each day.

Gone are the days that meditation is all 'woo-woo' and hippie. There is solid science in the number of benefits.

It can:

Increase your positive emotions (111, 112).

Decrease depression (113).

Decrease anxiety (114, 115).

Decrease stress (116, 117).

Increases immune function (118).

Decrease inflammation at a cellular level (119, 120).

Increases memory and ability to focus and attention (121, 122, 123).

Do what you enjoy:

The third step is to do what you enjoy.

It amazed me when I first discovered this myself, listening to a Tony Robbins talk where he was listing all the things he loves. The actions that bring him joy, and how I first had no real idea of what I enjoyed. And secondly, how I didn't focus on doing more of these things.

So, start with simply listing out what are the top five things that bring you joy.

It could be spending time with friends, listening to music, going for a surf, painting, or having a hard, kickboxing workout.

Whatever it is, plan to do at least two of these things a day.

Movement: The Yin and the Yang

We've already covered in the Training for Fat Loss chapter, how we can break up your exercise and movement into three basic components. The truth is, though, that I just want you to move your body. So many health and fitness professionals are caught up with having a totally optimal program design, that they forget that you're a busy human being, living a life.

Yes, if you follow the workouts I've designed for you, you're going to be able to accelerate your fat loss. But I know, that many reading this can just flat out NOT like to exercise, or specifically, not like to lift weights.

This can happen because maybe you've had a bad experience before, and you're scared. Maybe you're scared of going into a new environment like the gym that many perceive as 'scary' or 'intimidating.' I understand that, because that's how I felt when I first walked into a gym in my late teens. Though looking back, I was scared and intimidated because I didn't know what to do.

And that's why I want to give you the plans to follow, which also include the videos and guides in the Free Download site you get access to with this book, so that you can walk into the gym and have confidence in knowing what and how to train.

The truth is, though, if you love Zumba (or any other type of movement and exercise), then that is fantastic. And I want you to have a strong relationship combining exercise and enjoyment.

The fact that you have to sweat and push yourself physically is a trait that is built upon step-by-step. I remember having clients that first joined a gym, where I would literally hold their hand and walk them into the free weights part of the gym. They had only ever been in the cardio section with the treadmills and bikes. Having taken, for example, a woman in her mid-thirties who was petrified of sweating and physical exertion, to doing a full chin up all by herself.

It's not the physical transformation that impresses me, it's the personal transformation. It's seeing men and women change how they walk, hold themselves, their confidence, and then their ability to go out and in life and use the experience and personal growth that stemmed from their training to bring into so many other aspects of their life.

This is why I believe that movement and training should be a part of all our lives. In our modern lifestyles, we're simply sitting too much. Personally, I had a really hard time transitioning from personal training clients and being in the gym, constantly moving to being in a home office, sitting at my desk for hours at a time.

This is why I love walking, as it just gets me out and about, moving. Stimulating my body and brain. But also, why there is a real need for our bodies to move. The gym and your training is the 'dojo' that gives you the ability to build your body and your health.

Sleep and Wind Down (just chill out more).

I started this chapter with sleep for a very good reason.

It's a simple and super effective way for you to reduce and manage stress, and allow your body to optimize itself. And rather than just telling you to "sleep more," like so much of the mainstream media barks at you, it is far more effective to look at the quality of your sleep first.

This is why we start with a Wind Down Routine, to set yourself up for rejuvenating sleep.

After guide-pigging this out on myself for months, and then testing and trialing different protocols with clients, we've used sleep tracking apps to see improvements in the restfulness and a greater quality of sleep that a Wind Down Routine can do for you.

Being able to avoid the tossing and turning, and "monkey mind" keeping you awake, you can fall asleep quickly, and be able to drop into the deep REM sleep that truly brings about beneficial changes.

We start with three simple steps to creating your Wind Down Routine.

1. Switch off your electronics, phone, computer, and TV.

Starting with 30 minutes before you go to bed, "it's time to get away from your TV, to stop scrolling through social media, and to allow the blue light of electronics to stop stimulating your brain.

The secret for this is to have a replacement. So instead of the usual routine of what you're currently doing before going to bed, let's replace it with reading, stretching, meditation, taking a bath, or just chilling out and talking with a loved one.

For my wife, Lauren, and me, it's usually a few candles, herbal tea, and chatting about life.

Also, this is can dramatically help your sex life.

If you're in the routine of slouching on the couch for an hour, then dragging yourself to bed when you know it's getting late, don't expect to suddenly burst into a romantic and intimate scene.

Pro Tip: I understand that you can't always get away from this, especially if you have to work sometimes. For example, I interview some people for the podcast either super early or later, after my bedtime. I use an app on my mac called Flux that can take the blue light out of your screen, to lower the stimulation of the brain perceived through the eyes.

2. Upgrade What You Eat and Drink Before Bed.

There certainly are nutrients that can help you wind down and set you up for a great sleep.

This is one reason magnesium is a part of a complete

supplement stack, as it's a very common deficient as it's so asking from the foods we eat.

Magnesium is the only supplement that I'll talk about here, as when you join us in the My Body Blends community, there are episodes and guides that go deeper into this to individualize it for you. Also, the most important parts are the foods, drink, and lifestyle factors you can take first.

We talked about in the debunking of the "you should eat carbs at the start of the day," how eating carbohydrates at the end of the day can have many beneficial effects. One being, helping you to sleep. You'll find that after the 14-Day Metabolic Switch phase of the My Body Diet, we start to include more starchy carbohydrates to your diet, and we place it as the last meal of the day.

This is because it can influence greater relaxation and mood elevation. The carbohydrates can help you produce serotonin, a key neurotransmitter that is best known as the "feel good" brain chemical, which helps provide a sense of calm. The carbs also help lower cortisol, which aids your body following the natural cycle of cortisol secretion, which is high in the morning and low at night. This happens because the carbs help produce insulin, which is an antagonist to cortisol.

Lastly, we know after the last chapter on the Inner Game, that willpower has a shellfire and not something that you want to rely on when it comes to sticking to a diet or weight loss program. Through experience, I've found the vast majority of people prefer eating carbs at night, and they can sustain the willpower to eat the foods they want to and not overeat when using this method.

Personally, I am busy through the days. I use my foods to fuel my brain and my body and can happily see food as fuel during the entire day. This is why I focus on protein, vegetables, and fats in a more metabolic state for the daytime. But dinner is the meal where I want to sit and enjoy: Both with my friends and family, and where I really take stock for the day and have a larger meal. So my dinners are when I will eat more overall compared to my other meals, and where I eat most of my carbohydrates.

Then, as also mentioned above, we enjoy an herbal tea to help us wind down. Chamomile has properties that will help with sleep, there are many great tea mixtures that are specially formulated for helping you sleep. However, I personally just like peppermint or ginger tea to finish the day.

3. Prepare the 'Bat Cave.'

The bedroom, I believe, is for two things… Sleep and sex.

There should be no phones, TV's, or electronics in your bedroom. The room should be pitch black, first taking out electronics from the room saves you from pituitary stimulating little blinking lights that can come from chargers, phones, or that little red light on your TV when it's turned off.

Using blackout shades for your blinds is a great help here, as the light that can sneak in from your windows and even doors can still stimulate or disturb your sleep.

Secondly, there should be no noise. Now, if you're living alongside a busy road (compared to our current home being next to a rice paddy), ear plugs are going to be the easiest option. As the goal here is to create a 'bat cave.' A cool, dark, quiet place that gives you a superb sleeping environment.

Then, it's best to have a cool temperature for your room. In general, the suggested bedroom temperature should be between 60 and 67 degrees Fahrenheit for optimal sleep.

Now that we have covered the two key factors of lifestyle being sleep and stress, let's go onto the fourth key pillar for your body and health.

After interviewing over 100 of the world's top experts, it was when I had the pleasure of talking to Jay Ferruggia on the show, was one of the moments where I was sitting face to face with someone that I have highly respected and learned from for many years.

And every time, these world-leading experts keep coming back the basics. It's because they are the most important. So much of the confusion and conflicting information are in the large number of books, blogs, and videos. Jay graciously shared the key steps to why he's able to impact and transform so many bodies around the world for decades, and continues to do so.

It's his advice that concerted in just how I had to structure this book and the programs to ensure you get the easiest, fastest, and longest lasting results.

32
SUPPLEMENTS

The Truth to What Supplements WORK

Have you ever walked into a sports supplement store and felt overwhelmed and confused?

The sheer number of different products for you to choose from.

The U.S. weight loss market totaled $64 billion in 2014 according to Marketdata Enterprises. And it's continuing to grow.

Then there are all the outrageous marketing claims being made. All while you are just trying to figure out "what is best for me?"

Most of the products lining the shelves at your local supplement store are packed full of ineffective ingredients that are NOT backed by any real scientific research… they're typically under-dosed, poorly formulated, and have the specific ingredient amounts hidden behind "proprietary blends"… and in some cases, they don't even actually contain what the label says.

Supplements are just that… to supplement your whole food diet.

This is why, even as a founder and owner of a company that sells whole food supplements, the entire concept of My Body Blends is to first have you eat, move, and live in a way that has you looking, feeling, and functioning the way you want. And then combining it with the whole food supplements that support everything you're doing.

As the Standard American Diet (SAD) shifts further and further away from nutrient-dense foods like high-quality, animal protein and vegetables, nutrient deficiency is becoming a widespread epidemic.

But even if you're following a more nutrient-dense diet full of quality protein and fats, you can no longer rely on getting all your nutrients from food.

Why We "Need" Nutritional Supplements

In a perfect world, no one would need supplements. But given the stress of our modern life, the poor quality of our food supply, and the high load of toxins in our brains and bodies, most of us need a basic daily supply of the raw materials for all our enzymes and biochemistry to run as designed.

For years, I was always thinking of different vitamins and minerals and how they all work in isolation: The thoughts of, "I just need more magnesium," so take more magnesium supplements any time of the day. However, this was flawed thinking.

For example, zinc, magnesium, calcium, and iron all compete for transporters in the intestine for uptake. So taking them at the same time, could be ineffective. And Another example is how too much zinc supplementation can lead to a copper deficiency.

We can get so focused on the health benefits of a certain vitamin or phytochemical that we miss an important point: Different components in a single food can work together to benefit our health, and so can components in different foods that are eaten together.

This brings us to the importance of 'food synergy' and how foods and nutrients need to work together. David Jacobs, PhD, a researcher from the University of Minnesota, loosely defines food synergy as the idea that food influences our health in complex and highly interactive ways. The Produce for Better Health Foundation explains it as nutrients working together to create greater health effects.

The ability of a vitamin or mineral to be used by our body is called bioavailability. The bioavailability of a nutrient depends on its efficiency in digestion, foods eaten at the same meal, the way the food was prepared, and whether the vitamin is natural, synthetic, or fortified in foods.

Vitamins and minerals often work together to perform different functions in the body. For example, vitamin D regulates calcium balance, and these nutrients work together to affect bone mass. Vitamin C assists in the absorption of iron, which is essential for prevention of anemia. Thus, our intake of certain nutrients affects not only the body's ability to maintain levels of other nutrients, but also, the ability of the body to perform essential functions. In this three-part series, we will learn about how vitamins and minerals affect our health and wellbeing.

First of all, grains, legumes, and conventional dairy are low in nutrients and difficult for a lot of people to digest. Grains and legumes contain phytic acid and other compounds that can interfere with nutrient absorption and can cause intestinal damage, which makes it even harder for your body to absorb nutrients [144, 145, 146, 147, 148]. Even if you've stopped eating these foods, you may be in nutrient debt or have lingering intestinal damage, which is interfering with nutrient absorption. Dairy, especially conventional dairy, is inflammatory and difficult to digest for many people. It also contains mycotoxins which are extremely inflammatory [149].

Then there is the problem of our soil depletion…

Improper farming practices deplete the soil of essential nutrients. When plants are repeatedly grown on the same land, the soil loses vitamins, minerals, and microbes faster than they can be replaced. Over time, the plants have fewer nutrients to grow. Fertilizer contains just enough nutrition for the plant to survive until harvesting, but not enough to support human health. In addition, most plants are not eaten when fresh. They sit on trucks, shelves, and counters for weeks before being eaten. Over time, the nutrient content of these plants decreases.

Most modern fruits and vegetables are grown to increase their sugar content, not their nutrient value [150]. As a result, the most common fruits and vegetables are artificially high in fructose and lower in key nutrients [151].

When plants contain fewer nutrients, the animals that eat these plants are also malnourished. A study published in the Journal of Nutrition and Health found copper levels in the UK have dropped 90% in dairy, 55% in meat, and 76% in vegetables [152]. Copper is an essential nutrient that helps to regulate several pathways in the body, including energy production and brain function [153].

After soil depletion, there is the issue of water depletion...

Water is also depleted of minerals due to modern production methods. There is a huge variation in the mineral content of bottled and tap water, with tap water generally having more [154].

Agronomist Phil Warman says that modern farming practices and market emphasis are mostly at fault for nutrient degradation. According to his research, "The emphasis is on appearance, storability, and transportability, and there has been much less emphasis on the nutritional value of fruits and vegetables." "High-yield production and disease-resistance are much more important to food producers today," says Warman, "than nutritional content of foods."

The entire process from poor soil where the food is grown to the farming methods used, to how it's manufactured and processed and the effects of long-term food storage, as well as the effects of improper cooking and heating of foods can destroy the nutrients. One of the best resources I recommend is the book, Nourishing Traditions, by Sally Fallon. We're releasing the new My Body Cookbook to walk you through how to easily shop, prepare, cook, and enjoy meals that are richest in nutrients.

Now, if you're like me and many of my clients and members,

you've tried the low-calorie approach before.

There is no doubt that the My Body Diet is designed to fuel you with nutrient-rich meals you enjoy. As humans, we're designed to consume large amounts of nutrient-dense calories to meet our body's needs [155]. When you're constantly restricting your caloric intake, it's easy to become malnourished.

Animal foods are generally higher in calories and nutrients, so it's no surprise that's where the majority of calories came from in early human development [156]. Since the modern trend is to reduce the consumption of animal foods, people are consuming fewer nutrients per unit of food [157].

Then there is the debate of organic versus non-organic foods and whether there is a real health benefit.

There is research, and where my view currently stands, that organic is the superior option.

Non-organic, pesticide-treated vegetables are lower in cancer-fighting polyphenols than organic ones. This is because the plant produces polyphenols as a defense against bugs and pathogens. When there is no reason to defend themselves, the plant stops producing polyphenols, and your body and brain suffer the consequences [158].

One of the big issues I see with non-organic food is the evidence that glyphosate – RoundUp herbicide – chelates minerals in crops on which it is sprayed. It remains to be seen how much of an impact this effect has, but it's safe to avoid GMO foods for a variety of other reasons [159].

Then there are the modern lifestyle stresses and toxins that we all go through each day.

Your body needs nutrients to deal with toxins. When more toxins are present, you need more nutrients.

Pesticides, herbicides, and chemicals found in the modern food supply are combined with chemicals in water, environmental contamination from elements such as degraded plastic, air pollution from carbon monoxide, lead and mercury. These synergistic elements vastly increase our need for extra vitamins, minerals, and nutrients to combat the formation of free radicals and the attack upon our metabolism and immune system.

Here are just some of the things your body has to contend with:

1. Xenoestrogens (plastics, BPA, some molds, petroleum products).
2. Industrial solvents and cleaners.
3. Unnatural lighting.
4. Food toxins (not a problem if you're eating Bulletproof).
5. Stress and lack of sleep.

And it's my belief, and by learning from so many of the world's best when it comes to this, (especially the teachings I've had from Dr. Bob Rokwaski and Dr. Mark Schuss) that there is a real need for nutritional aid to help the body thrive.

Then, there is the factor of ease.

For example, I love salmon. However, the cost and ease for me to be able to use a high-quality fish oil supplement that isn't laden with chemicals make it an easy option for me to take. This doesn't replace me eating salmon or fish. It just means that I can get the amount of Omega 3's that I want, easily.

Farmed salmon is low in Omega-3s and high in toxins [160]. Farmed salmon are higher in parasites and bacteria. To hide the sickly appearance of farmed salmon meat, the fish are fed a pink pigment to change their tissue color. Farmed salmon contains 16 times more PCB's and pesticides than the wild version [161].

Are you actually absorbing the nutrients?

Once food makes it past your mouth and is swallowed down past your esophagus, the acid wash inside the stomach begins, and not surprisingly, another host of problems can start to occur. The environment inside your stomach is highly acidic (pH 4), and this acid acts as the next defense mechanism against harmful pathogens that might have slipped past your first line of defense. A protective mucous lining protects your stomach from all this acid.

When I talk about acids in your stomach, I am referring to hydrochloric acid and pepsin. Compromised stomach acidity is a common hindrance to optimum digestion, and can frequently be aided by supplementing with hydrochloric acid (Betaine HCL) or digestive enzymes.

This is why your gut health is so important and why compromised gut health can lead to you not digesting, absorbing, or assimilating the foods and nutrients so you can make use of them.

I love the idea that you can get all your nutrients from food. The theory makes me warm and fuzzy. However, the realistic nature of our modern lifestyles means that we are not able to eat the foods that are rich in the nutrients we need. And then there are all the factors, such as soil and water depletion, food and environmental toxins, poor absorption, pesticides, exercise, and lack of calories that can all cause nutrient deficiencies. There is evidence that consuming nutrients from food is more beneficial than supplements, which is why you should focus on a nutrient-rich diet first [162]. However, it's rarely enough anymore.

The question I want answered for you is not, "how much of a certain nutrient or vitamin you need to avoid illness," but "how much you need to be optimally healthy?"

Dr. Robert Heaney, one of the world's leading vitamin D researchers, in a recent groundbreaking editorial in The American Journal of Clinical Nutrition about the delayed (yet very serious) consequences of taking LESS than the optimal amounts of nutrients for life said, "because the current [vitamin] recommendations are based on the prevention of the [deficiency] disease only, they can no longer be said to be biologically defensible. The pre-agricultural human diet ... may well be a better starting point for policy. The burden of proof should fall on those who say that these more natural conditions are not needed and that lower intakes [of nutrients] are safe."

Why We Start with Quality over Quantity...

There are three things in life I see when we should NOT skimp and worry about price;

1. Parachutes... You don't want this malfunctioning.

2. Tattoos… They are on you for life!

3. Supplements… You need the quality and potency to get the results and effects you want.

Yes, this is a little tongue in cheek. But this is just an example of "you get what you pay for." Though you have to ask yourself, "what's the point of choosing something cheap if you don't even get the result you want?"

And with the supplement industry, it's filled with smoke and mirrors, with a thick number of lies that you have to cut through. It was a huge motivating factor for me to start My Body Blends and want to go toe-to-toe with the supplement giants. Personally, I was sick and tired of being screwed over. Health and supplement stores, along with online retailers, are filled with countless options that are either made with inferior products or manufacturing standards. Or even worse, just plain lying about what is in the product. Recently, there have been 100s of companies that have been tested and found that their products DON'T have what they claim is on the label.

It is important to find safe, high-quality, and effective nutritional supplement products. Be aware that all brands are not created equally. Quality is up to the manufacturer because of limited regulations regarding manufacturing. Certain companies are more careful about quality, sourcing of raw materials, consistency of dose from batch to batch, the use of active forms of nutrients, not using fillers, additives, colorings, etc. When choosing supplements, it is important that you choose quality products.

We now know that there can be a need for effective nutritional supplements, now it's about answering, "what do you take to get the best results… and save yourself money?"

The Foundation Stack

The Foundation Stack is made of the three supplements that I believe are to be the best benefit, along with the biggest bang for your buck.

Fish Oil and Omega 3s

Fish oil can help you lose body fat for a number of reasons. Some are well known, while other reasons are still emerging. Omega 3 fatty acids are a part of the essential fats that our bodies can't create on their own, and therefore, need to get from our diet.

Studies show that when fish oil is included in a healthy lifestyle intervention, it can help to reduce waist circumference and decrease fat mass (137, 138).

It accomplishes this in several ways, including reducing appetite, improving circulation and thereby nutrient delivery to skeletal muscle, and augmenting muscle gain, which enhances fat oxidation and energy expenditure.

Fish oil provides your body with two nutrients that are otherwise hard to get enough of through diet alone:

Eicosatetraenoic acid (EPA)
Docosahexaenoic acid (DHA)

The reason it's a "thing" as far as supplementation goes is that the fats in these fish are a very good source of the nutrients mentioned above: EPA and DHA. You could just eat the fish, but you'd have to eat quite a bit every week to get enough of these vital nutrients.

Together, EPA and DHA are known as "Omega-3 fatty acids," which refers to their physical structure, and our bodies can't produce them, which is why they're also known as "essential fatty acids."

That is, if you were to completely remove these molecules from your diet, you would eventually die.

Unfortunately, studies show that the average person's diet provides just one-tenth of the EPA and DHA needed to preserve health and prevent disease (127).

Now, fatty fish aren't the only way to increase your EPA and DHA intake, grass-fed meat, free-range eggs, and vegetable oils are other sources.

Omega-3 levels are much lower in meat and eggs than fish, though, and vegetable oils don't contain EPA and DHA, but instead, contain a fatty acid called alpha-linolenic acid (ALA), which the body then converts into EPA and DHA.

The problem with ALA, however, is that the conversion process is very inefficient, so you would have to eat large amounts of ALA to supply your body with enough EPA and DHA.

Fish Oil Enables You Lose Fat and Build Muscle.

We've talked in-depth about the importance of insulin sensitivity, and fish oil allows this to be raised. It does this as it gets incorporated into the cellar lipid layer, which allows the cell receptors to bind more easily to the hormone, insulin. Because it can bind easily, it's able to do its job far more effectively, which is to shuttle glucose to the muscles to be stored, and used as energy later.

In this study (124), subjects took about 2 grams of Omega 3 fatty acids (EPA and DHA) every day for 6 weeks. At the end of the study, they had lost more than 2 lbs. of body fat. The subjects also gained about 1 pound of lean body mass.

You can also see fish oil working in a recent study (125) that gave subjects either 4 grams of fish oil, or 4 grams of safflower oil (a type of Omega 6 fat) for 6 weeks. The subjects that took the fish oil significantly lost more body fat and increased muscle tissue. And this is without even exercising.

Also, fish oil will help reduce inflammation, which significantly enhances your body's ability to lose body fat and build muscle (114).

Fish oil has also been shown to:

- Reduce the risk of heart disease, stroke and type 2 diabetes (129, 130, 131).
- Improve mood and brain health (132, 133).
- Help prevent weight gain (134).
- Help fat loss (135).
- Help muscle growth (136).

Research shows that 500mg to 1.8 grams of EPA and DHA per day can be effective. But additional health benefits can be seen up to a combined intake of 6 grams per day (126).

Greens Superfood

It's a well-known fact that people who eat higher amounts of fruits and vegetables are, on the whole, healthier and more likely to live longer, disease-free lives than those who don't eat enough.

This is why one of the main steps in most meals is to include the "all you can eat carbs" that are the nutrient-dense, fiber-dense vegetables.

Greens superfoods powder supplements have many question marks around them. What do they do? Are they worth it? and "What should I be having?

It's time you finally have the truth…

You will no longer be wasting away hundreds of dollars on pills and potions that you know don't make you feel any different, and you never see a change.

The confusion when it comes to knowing what supplements you need to be taking is something we know all too well. Walking into a sports nutrition store can be mind boggling; you have wall-to-wall choices and the person serving is usually overly excited, and never actually looking that healthy anyway… who do you listen to?

…and I get it.

Despite it being prostituted in the media, there is no official or legal definition of a superfood. The Oxford English dictionary, for example, describes a superfood as "a nutrient-rich food considered to be especially beneficial for health and wellbeing."

To distinguish the truth from the hype, it is important to look carefully at the scientific evidence behind the media's superfood claims. Blueberries are one of the more popular and well-known superfoods, and they have frequently been studied by scientists curious about their health properties. The berries' high concentrations of a group of antioxidant plant compounds, especially those called anthocyanins, have been reported to inhibit the growth of cancerous colon cells in humans, as well as kill them off.[5] Blueberries are also rich in other antioxidants, which have been shown to prevent and reverse age-related memory decline in rats.[6]

Antioxidants are molecules which protect the cells in the body from harmful free radicals. These free radicals come from sources such as cigarette smoke and alcohol, and they are also produced naturally in the body during metabolism. Too many free radicals in the body can result in oxidative stress, which in turn, causes cell damage that can lead to age-related diseases such as cancer, diabetes, and heart disease.[7]

One major characteristic of research in this area is that very high levels of nutrients tend to be used. These are usually not realistically attainable in the context of a normal diet. This is why at My Body Blends we poured through the research for countless hours to give you the perfect combination of easy to use and effectiveness to suit your everyday life.

The reason we include the greens superfood as a part of the Foundation Stack is because it's your 'nutritional safeguard.' It not only is your multivitamin, it also has your antioxidants, phytonutrients, and even pro biotics.

Although no magic supplement exists for weight loss, some evidence suggests that taking multivitamins may help you burn more calories. Getting adequate amounts of vitamins and minerals is vital for a proper metabolism. Metabolism is the chemical reaction that your body uses to turn the food you eat into energy. Some vitamins, such as the B vitamins, play an important role in metabolizing dietary carbohydrates, fats, and proteins.

A study was done looking at how multivitamins change cholesterol levels and weight in obese women (142). The goal was to see if taking multivitamins would change bodyweight, energy expenditure, and lipid profiles (cholesterol). There was no change in diet or exercise with the test subjects.

And on average, the multivitamin group: Lost 3.4 kgs (7.5lb) of weight, decreased their weight circumference by 2.4cm, and lost 2.8kg (6.1lb) of fat. The test subjects who took the multivitamin saw an increase in their resting energy expenditure. Plus, their respiratory quotient (RQ), which is used to figure out if you are burning more carbohydrate or fat for energy, went from 0.81 to 0.78, which means they were burning more fat at rest.

And whether you want more energy each day, slimming and re-shaping your body, or knowing you are nourishing your body with the right nutrients, it comes down to -

…"my health, is my responsibility."

This is the exact outcome I came to after years of following fad diets, mainstream advice, and being worse off from it. After going out and learning from the best in the world and spending countless hours, years even, researching what really works, I was able to put it to the test and see the changes within myself, my clients, and my members worldwide. It is my passion to give you the right advice, information, and guidance to empower you to get the body, health, and happiness we all want.

The truth is –

A greens superfood powder doesn't replace the power of a wholesome, nutrient-dense diet. A supplement is exactly that – it is a supplement to your diet.

Now, there is a big buzz around green juices, but to be honest, I'm not the biggest fan of these for everyday use. When you juice, you don't keep the pulp and fibrous material of the fruits and veggies (the good stuff). This is why I prefer smoothies.

However, the biggest benefit of juicing is the absorption of nutrients. Consuming a freshly pressed juice is like giving yourself a nutrient shot! The veggies are partially digested, your body can soak them up quickly. When you have the fibrous parts of the plants removed, and the cell walls are broken down, it allows your body's own enzymes to act on these nutrients with ease.

This is where a greens superfood powder drink comes in as my favorite choice. Your body can easily process and absorb the nutrients, and it is a perfect way to deliver the digestive aid blend and probiotics that I want in a Superfood Blend. It's been shown time and time again that your gut health is imperative to your overall health. So many hormones and neurotransmitters are created in the gut, it's been shown to be the 'second brain.'

Since greens supplements are vegetable powerhouses, it's been proposed that they're a good way to optimize your body's pH. They might actually work that way. A study published in the "Journal of the International Society of Sports Nutrition" found that two weeks of daily supplementation with greens led to significant improvements in urinary pH, moving subjects from an acidic pH to one considered optimal. The results from this pilot-type study suggest that a daily greens supplement may improve an acid-base balance that is out of the optimal range.

Some nutritional experts recommend consuming at least 60 percent of your diet as alkaline foods, and the remaining 40 percent as acid foods.

"Green superfoods" can help provide balance to your acid foods*. A few of the top alkaline-forming foods include vegetables, such as alfalfa, barley, wheatgrass, beets, broccoli, cabbage, kale, and spinach.

As for beverages, green tea is alkaline-forming, while coffee, alcohol, black tea, and any type of soda are acid-forming.

The many nutritional benefits that emerged from these extensive studies were credited to the grasses' supply of chlorophyll and vitamins. The most important nutrients in cereal grasses were found to be:

- Phytopigments such as chlorophyll and carotenoids
- The plant sterol ester, beta-sitosterol
- Antioxidants, such as superoxide dismutase and beta-carotene
- Vitamins B1, B2, B6, B12, pantothenic acid, and folic acid
- Potassium, calcium, iron, phosphorus, and magnesium

What it really boils down to, is that I wanted a total solution to today's less-than-optimal choices. I wanted a high-quality formula that would tick the boxes to give me what I needed:

- Quick and easy to use
- Easily taken with shakes, smoothies, and protein powder drinks
- Provide a simple way to get your nutrients with your protein
- No strong, unpleasant "green" taste
- …actually tastes really good
- Include nature's powerful superfoods loaded with vitamins and minerals
- Include the SuperVegetox Antioxidant and Fruit Antioxidant blend
- Provide a blend of digestive support and gut health
- Contain exceptional alkalizing extracts that provide antioxidant benefits
- Contain all tested non-GMO and gluten-free ingredients

And really knowing that in 30 seconds from mixing in water and drinking, it's the nutritional insurance that's nourishing my body.

For me having all of the above, gives me peace of mind that you will:

- Feel the difference in your energy by having the nutrients, enzymes, and co-factors you're not currently getting from your diet.

- Instead of wasting money on a cupboard full of poor-quality supplements, save hundreds by using this one, simple and powerful Superfood Blend.
- With 50 whole food ingredients, you are giving yourself nutritional insurance for a healthy future.
- Nutritionally aid your body's own detox system to clear out toxins that can cause illness and blunt the fat burning process.

Greens and Weight Loss

A research team in Kyoto, Japan found that chlorella promotes weight loss by controlling gene expression to produce reductions in body fat percentages, fasting glucose levels, and total circulating cholesterol (139). Researchers tracked two groups of participants; one at high risk for lifestyle-related disease, and one made up of healthy individuals. Their findings were consistent across both groups. Genes positively affected by chlorella included those related to signaling, transport, fat metabolism, glucose uptake, and insulin pathways.

Further, a research team in Korea has found that chlorella can actually make fat cells drop dead, while leaving other cells untouched. It can shrink fat cells too, by decreasing the amount of fat held within them. Chlorella can even rev up enzyme action in fat cells to produce energy and increase metabolism (140).

One animal study has highlighted chlorella for its use as a natural medicine against obesity-related complications that include irregularities in body weight, lipid profile, blood glucose, and insulin signaling. This study demonstrated that chlorella's prevention of diet-induced insulin resistance is at least in part due to its improvement in insulin signaling pathways. Researchers also found that chlorella reduces triglycerides, cholesterol, and free fatty acid levels (141).

This gives us a clear picture that for a nutritional safeguard, a quality superfood greens formula earns its place in the Foundation Stack.

How Probiotics Can Help with Weight Loss

From our modern diet to stress, age, exposure to environmental toxins, excessive hygiene, the overuse of antibiotics (both as medicine and in our food supply), as well as the frequent use of medicines like birth control, acid suppressants (PPIs), antacids, steroids, hormone replacement therapy, and NSAIDs, many of us have damaged the very system that is in place to protect and sustain us: our microbiome.

These living organisms have been credited with providing all kinds of health benefits related to gut function and beyond (169). Their functions include converting fiber into short-chain fatty acids, synthesizing certain vitamins, and supporting your immune system (170).

And as we talked about in the previous section, "How to Fix Your Gut Bacteria and Lose Weight," we now know that gut health has a strong influence on our body's ability to lose weight. As both human and animal studies have found that normal weight people have different gut bacteria than overweight or obese people (188,189).

And when we have an unhealthy gut, this can lead to poor nutrient absorption and digestion, as well as poor mental, metabolic, and immune function. Everything from your energy levels to your mood, mental state, and weight stems from the balance of good flora inside your GI tract.

So along with eating foods that are rich in prebiotics and probiotics, it's the probiotics that still make sense to supplement, and why we include them as a part of the Foundation Stack.

Though not all probiotics supplements are the same, as many of the probiotics supplements can be dead or just ineffective when you take them.

There are two big reasons why most probiotic supplements are ineffective…

1. The probiotic bacteria are dead by the time they get into your gut.

Probiotics are sensitive organisms. They die quickly when exposed to heat and moisture.

You see, we weren't meant to need probiotic supplementation in the first place--because we weren't meant to damage our microbiome. But since we have, it's now vital that we repopulate our digestive tracts, and the only way to do this effectively is to ensure that the beneficial bacteria make it past the stomach acids alive, so that they can colonize in our small and large intestine, where we actually need them.

The problem is that, without protection, most of the bacteria in probiotic supplements are killed before they ever reach their destination.

2. They don't deliver the sufficient variety of strains or potency

We believe that to be effective, probiotic supplementation should deliver a variety of strains to properly counter these indiscriminate effects. Each strain performs a different function within the intestinal tract and offers a different set of benefits to the individual.

Because the different strains of probiotic bacteria have slightly different functions and are concentrated in various places along the digestive tract, probiotic supplements that contain multiple strains tend to be more effective overall than products containing an extremely high concentration of just one or two strains. This is because many strains work synergistically to influence our health. The whole, literally, is greater than the sum of its parts.

In addition, it's important to consume probiotics in sufficient amounts.

Probiotics are typically measured in colony-forming units (CFU). Generally, higher doses have been found to produce the best results in most studies (171).

Some studies suggest that taking probiotic supplements may be helpful for achieving weight loss and a healthier body composition. There is growing evidence that the balance of bacteria in your gut can profoundly affect body weight (172).

Animal and human studies have found that certain bacterial

strains may decrease the amount of fat and calories your gut absorbs, promote a healthy balance of gut bacteria, and reduce weight and belly fat (173, 174, 175, 176, 177, 178).

In one study, obese men who took L. gasseri for 12 weeks experienced significant reductions in body weight and body fat, including up to an 8.5% decrease in belly fat. By contrast, the placebo group had very little change in body weight or body fat (179).

And as you know, I'm a firm believer in the connection between our brains and bodies, and how we need to promote health to both. The bacteria in your colon digest and ferment fiber into short-chain fatty acids that nourish the gut. Research has shown that these compounds may also benefit the brain and nervous system (180).

There are numerous studies that show probiotics have positively impacted anxiety, depression, autism, obsessive-compulsive disorder, poor memory, anxiety, sadness in healthy individuals and people with chronic fatigue syndrome. And taking probiotic supplements also appears to help people struggling with depression, including those with major depressive disorder, as well as showing reductions in insulin levels and inflammatory markers (181, 182, 183, 184, 185, 186).

The Truth to Fiber Supplements for Weight Loss

Honestly…

It's the synergy of the whole foods you eat that give you the best benefits. This is why getting your fiber firstly from whole plant foods is best, and then, looking to supplements as the answer.

As when you take isolated fibers extracted from plants, you're going to have a limited effect. Glucomannan is one fiber extracted from the Konjac root that has some evidence for showing benefits for weight loss when used as a supplement (163, 164, 165).

According to a report[17] by the Council for Responsible Nutrition Foundation (CRNF), if American adults over the age of 55 with heart disease took psyllium dietary fiber daily, it could reduce health care costs by nearly $4.4 billion a year (166).

This is exactly why we break down the My Body Diet to give you a broad range of foods rich in soluble and insoluble fiber. Including the viscous fibers exclusively found in plant foods.

Also, let's not forget that health is about way more than just weight. Eating plenty of fiber from real foods can have numerous other health benefits.

What many fail to realize is that grain-based fiber is far from ideal, as the grains that accompany it can actually promote insulin and leptin resistance.

Many whole foods, especially fruits and vegetables, naturally contain both soluble and insoluble fiber. This is ideal, as both help feed the microorganisms living in your gut. The same cannot be said for grains (including whole grains) and processed foods, as the carbohydrates found in both, can serve as fodder for microorganisms that tend to be detrimental to health. Gliadin and lectins in grains may also increase intestinal permeability or leaky gut syndrome.

Eating leafy greens such as spinach and kale, and vegetables in the cruciferous family, such as broccoli, cauliflower, cabbage, and bok-choy have several properties that make them great to include in your weight loss diet.

Eating these is a great way to increase the volume of your meals without increasing the calories. Numerous studies show that meals and diets with a low energy density make people eat fewer calories overall (167).

Leafy greens are also incredibly nutritious and very high in all sorts of vitamins, minerals, and antioxidants. This includes calcium, which has been shown to aid fat burning in some studies (168).

The key factor determining the fat-loss effects of fiber has to do with the amount of sugar/starch in a food compared to the amount of fiber. If a food is almost all sugar/starch and has very little fiber, blood sugar levels will surge, leading to energy swings that can cause changes in mood, food cravings, and hunger. However, if a food has a higher proportion of fiber compared to sugar/starch, the exact opposite is true, creating energy levels that are more stable, reduced cravings, and decreased hunger.

How Protein Can Help You Lose Weight and Belly Fat

The reality, though, is there is no such thing as a "weight loss food."

That said, certain foods are more conducive to weight loss than others.

The reason why some foods are "better" for weight loss than others, boils down to the number of calories they contain, and how those calories break down into protein, carbohydrate, and fat. And how these foods have a hormonal impact. This is why I include the fantastic interview with Dr. Bob Rakowski in the Bonus Downloads section under the title, "Food is more than just calories."

In broad strokes, the best foods for weight loss are those that provide you with an abundance of micronutrients, are filling, and help balance blood sugars. The foods you want to avoid when dieting (to lose weight) are those that are very calorie dense and high in dietary fat and added sugar, but which aren't all that filling.

Protein is the first macronutrient we focus on when putting your meals together. As protein is not only going to provide the essential building blocks (amino acids) for your body, it's also going to help boost your metabolism and have you burn slightly more calories each day (190,191).

It can also help decrease hunger and appetite in two ways.

First, by increasing levels of appetite-reducing hormones like GLP-1, PYY, and CCK, while reducing levels of the hunger hormone ghrelin (192, 193, 194). And secondly, protein can help you feel fuller for longer (195, 196).

Traditional weight loss diets often cause you to lose muscle, which can slow down your metabolism. This makes it easier to gain all the weight back (and more) once you stop the diet.

So, there is no doubt that we want to focus on the whole foods we eat to provide us with the vast majority of the protein we take in each day. However, over the past 12 years of coaching people around the world, literally, 1,000s have opted to include a protein shake during the day to hit their protein intake.

However, I'm not the biggest fan of just scooping some whey protein in water, then shaking and slamming it down. This isn't about sprinting to your locker immediately after the last set of your workout to skull down your protein shake in the hope of elevating your muscle growth and speeding up fat loss.

Much of the time, it's the ease and speed that you can enjoy a shake that provides you with a good dose of protein, along with nutrients that keep you fueled throughout the day. This is why you'll find in the recipes section, and especially in the Bonus Downloads, the recipes that we use with protein powders for shakes.

Honestly, you can easily get enough protein without using shakes. That being said, these supplements are an easy, safe, and enjoyable way to add extra protein in your diet.

If you're trying to lose weight, it's shown that extra protein from shakes can help you feel less hungry, help you lose weight faster, and lower the likelihood of regaining the lost fat.

Then it comes down to choosing the right protein powder. And if you're like me, you want one that:

- Is high in protein and low in added carbs and fats. As far as I'm concerned, any carbohydrate and fat in a protein powder are just "wasted" calories that I'd rather be eating.

- Has a minimal amount of added artificial sweeteners and fillers.
- Mixes well and tastes great, so you can enjoy each shake.
- Is well priced, so you're not wasting your money.

For me, I can be a delicate little snowflake, and my stomach doesn't tolerate the common whey protein very well. Even with the highly refined forms of whey, such as whey isolate or whey hydrolysate, which have virtually all lactose removed, I don't feel great after it, so therefore, avoid it.

Rather, opting for a vegan blend of protein so my digestion can happily absorb the protein, and also have the amino acids profile needed to be an effective protein supplement.

Non-soy sources of vegan protein, such as rice, hemp, and pea protein are often demonized as being "incomplete" and inferior sources of protein.

That is, some "experts" claim that these plant proteins are missing essential amino acids that your body needs, and thus, must be combined in special ways to form "complete" proteins that your body can use to build muscle and repair tissues.

What is true, however, is that some forms of vegan protein are <u>lower</u> in certain amino acids than others, and some are better absorbed by the body, making certain sources smarter choices than others.

This is why I'd rather a blend that can include rice, pea, and hemp protein.

Why You Need to 'Test' Yourself

There is no doubt that your body, compared to mine, needs different foods, nutrients, training, sleep, environment, and all the other factors to burn fat, to be in great health and thrive.

When it comes to supplementation, this chapter can easily become a whole book. And that's why I wanted to focus only on the Foundation Stack, including the importance of fiber. However, I could not just leave it here, as there are well researched, proven to work supplements and nutrients that you also "may" need.

And this is where the importance of testing comes in to play. You only know what it is you need if you find out what is lacking in your body.

For example, vitamin D is critically important to the body.

When I was personal training in Dubai, every single client that I referred to go get their blood work done came back with low vitamin D levels. At first, I was trying to figure out why. We were living in the middle of the dessert, and it's hot all year round. However, that was the problem. Because it is so hot in Dubai so much of the year, no one was getting out and getting sunlight exposure.

Then there is magnesium.

Magnesium is found in more than 300 different enzymes in your body and plays a role in your body's detoxification processes, making it important for helping to prevent damage from environmental chemicals, heavy metals, and other toxins. In addition, magnesium is necessary for:

- Activating muscles and nerves.
- Creating energy in your body by activating adenosine triphosphate (ATP).
- Helping digest proteins, carbohydrates, and fats.
- Serving as a building block for RNA and DNA synthesis.
- Acting as a precursor for neurotransmitters, such as serotonin.

By some estimates, up to 80 percent of Americans are not getting enough magnesium and may be deficient. Other research shows only about 25 percent of US adults are getting the recommended daily amount of 310 to 320 milligrams (mg) for women and 400 to 420 for men (143).

However, most foods grown today are deficient in magnesium and other minerals, so getting enough isn't simply a matter of eating magnesium-rich foods (although this is important too). According to Dr. Dean, who wrote The Magnesium Miracle:

"Magnesium is farmed out of the soil much more than calcium… A hundred years ago, we would get maybe 500 milligrams of magnesium in an ordinary diet. Now we're lucky to get 200 milligrams."

This is why I include in the Free Downloads and Guides section, the guide that helps you to know what testing you can easily and cheaply start with. So that you can have a personalized plan that nourishes your body to what it needs.

33
HOW TO GET IN THE BEST SHAPE OF YOUR LIFE

The 14-Day Metabolic Switch.

There's no better feeling than knowing your diet is working…

If you're like me and the other members I coach…

You're busy, and you want a plan that's simple to follow.

That's why in this chapter, I'm going to show you how we speed up weight loss with the best starting plan that kick starts you to faster results.

Even better, we're going to go through how to happily eat each meal using the **Metabolic Switch** as a starting meal plan for you.

As the truth is… You and I are busy.

You can't…
- Waste time consuming more information.
- Turn your life upside down trying to change a bunch of different things with your diet and lifestyle.

This is why I give you small, bite-sized steps only when you need it.

The entire plan is meticulously crafted so you have the simplest plan that evolves with you.

The 14-Day Metabolic Switch™ is simply made into 4-steps.

#1 - The Jump Start
#2 - The Fat Furnace
#3 - The Carb-Cycle
#4 - The Cleanse

We start with the 14-day jump start meal plan, so you will quickly throw each meal together in just 3-steps.

Your workouts can be in the gym or home, and you'll be spending less than 4 hours each week training.

And, importantly, I'll be showing you the lifestyle hacks that help turn your body into a fat-burning machine.

In each of the 4-phases of the Metabolic Switch™, we will focus on a key factor that ignites your metabolism and boosts your health.

Phase 1: The Jump Start

Let's go through the 4 easy steps right now to get you started…

The 14-Day Jump Start Meal Plan

1. Your Meal Plan

Put together each meal using these simple choices.

And no, I'm not worried about "how much" you are eating. If you get hungry, enjoy another meal. It's all about the food choices during these first 14-days.

The basic guidelines are:

- Decide on your 8-hour eating window. This stays the same for each day.
- Eat as much meat, poultry, eggs, and fish as you want in each meal.
- Eat unlimited vegetables from the "All You Can Eat Carbs List"
- http://mybodyblends.com/the-all-you-can-eat-carb-list/
- Include smart fats in your meals - Coconut oil, olive oil, avocado, butter.
- Eliminate all grains, potatoes, rice, pasta, cereals, and other starches.
- Eliminate dairy.
- Coffee can be black or Bulletproof (MCT oil and butter added)
- Drink 3L+ water each day.
- Salt EVERY meal (Himalayan pink salt and sea salt are great choices).

Leave a 2-hour gap between your last meal and bed.

Pro Tip:

We love green smoothies... Aim for 1x a day.

Use this super simple guide:

http://mybodyblends.com/superfood-green-smoothie-for-weight-loss/

2. Choose Your Eating Window.

This is a version of 'intermittent fasting,' but made for busy people living real lives.

Choose an 8-hour window in which you will eat your meals.

For example, I eat my first meal at 12pm midday, and finish my last meal at 8pm.

3. Take your "before" photo TODAY!

We need to track your changes. So please get someone to take your photo.

Guys wear underwear.

Gals wear a sports bra and underwear/shorts.

Please don't try and "suck it in," as we want a real snapshot of where you are.

4. Your Workouts

Schedule in 4x workouts each week.

Every day, you are also to go for at least a 30min walk... Have this in your calendar and planned.

I have the workout programs coming, but we have included it

in the free downloads section for you to have everything handy and mobile.

So, let's walk you through a common scenario that a lot of successful members have used.

- They chose to eat between 11am and 7pm.
- First meal at 11am was a green smoothie (Recipe in downloads section)
- They ate 3 other meals following the P-V-F meal model.
- Their last meal was at 7pm and was finished with a ginger and turmeric tea. That starts off their Wind Down Routine. More on this soon, as it's a part of our secret sauce for fast fat loss.

After the 14-Day Jump Start…
We then move onto the next steps being:

#2 - The Fat Furnace
#3 - The Carb-Cycle
#4 - The Cleanse

Once we complete the 4th and final week of the 14-Day Metabolic Switch™, we have an 11-step program that works with you month-to-month.

This is why we created the Bonus Section you can sign up for now to get the most out of having this book. So we can help give you the steps you need, when you need it. Just go to http://cravingthetruth.com/bookbonus.

This is exactly what Chaz used that got him started to lose 13 kilos of fat in just 10 weeks…

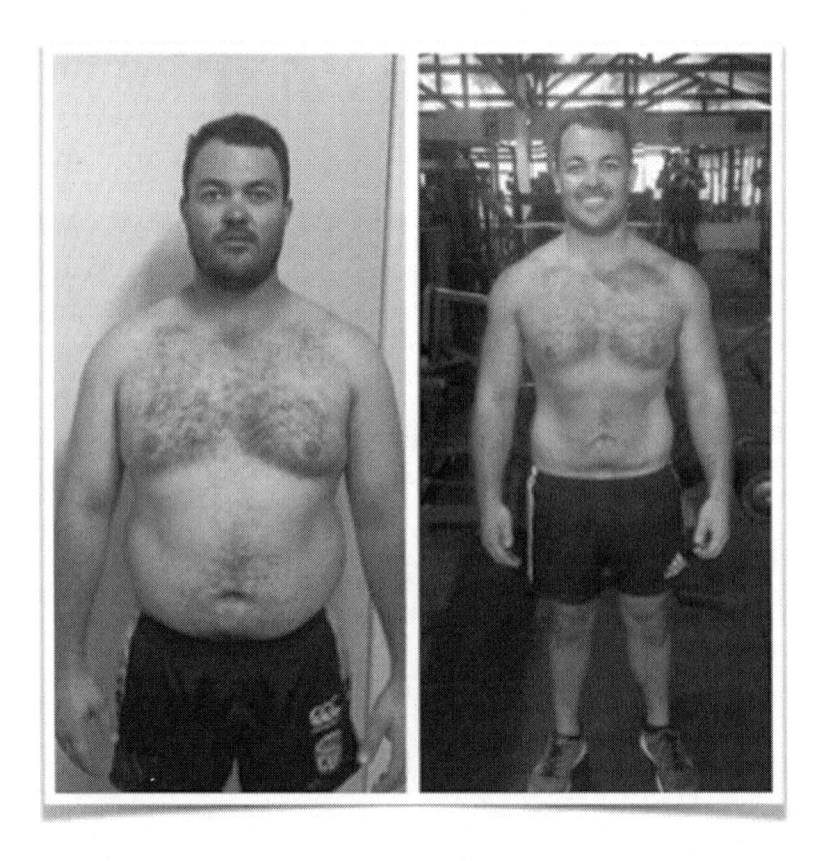

Also Michael, who transformed his physique, but did so with a crazy travel and work schedule…

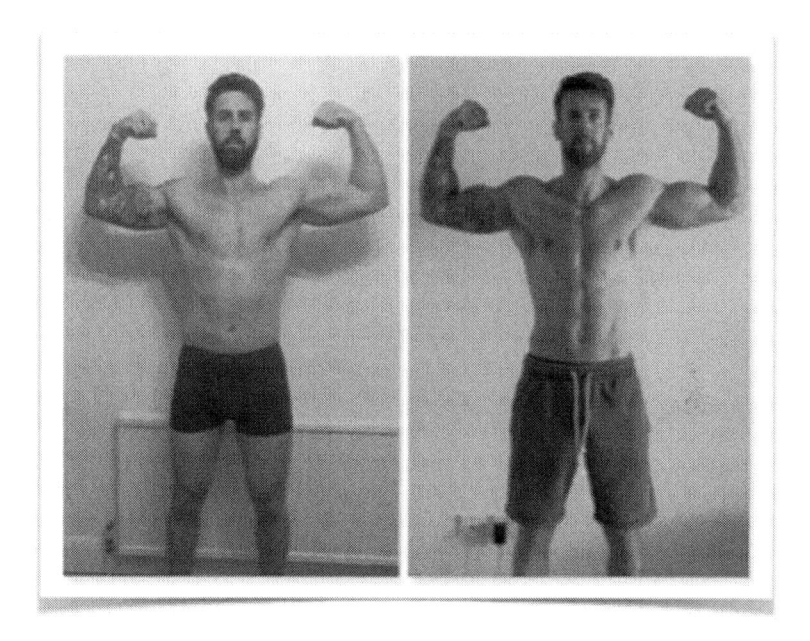

The 14-Day Metabolic Priming Phase

Phase 1 is the PERFECT 14-day cycle to start because it RESETS your body's fat burning switch by turning OFF your addiction to burning sugars, while reprogramming your body to use fat FIRST every time you eat and move.

This is known as becoming "FAT ADAPTED." And once you make the switch, they'll be no turning back.

The 14-Day Metabolic Switch serves several essential metabolic purposes that will reprogram your metabolism for long-term fat loss.

This jumpstart is essential for your success because it serves as the springboard that will move you through the flowing cycles. You'll automatically look and feel leaner, while you'll visually SEE your belly get flatter in just the first few days.

As let's be honest – you've probably already tried all the diets and been training hard – and it hasn't worked for you.

You want quick results… you don't want to slog through another diet, only to see mediocre (if any) results.

But, at the same time as your coach, it's my job to make sure we set you up for long-term success.

Firstly, this is super simple to follow.

A lot of people laugh at how simple it looks. They are expecting an elaborate meal plan with numbers and multiple pages to bring about amazing results.

> **Lindsay Brewer** 'TRUTH' by far the easiest meal plan I've ever followed 👍
> Like · Reply · 16 hrs

> **Kenneth Marafu**
> Hi Chris, your P-V-F Meal Plan of yours is ingenious. It is simple, easy and affordable. Just been following it for a week and I'm already seeing some great results. Feeling great man.
> Thanks a million

It's the simplicity wrapped in hormonal changes that makes this so powerful.

And that's why I DON'T want you counting calories or weighing your foods.

Science shows that everything to do with you burning fat is NOT just about calories. It's also the hormonal changes you can make with your meal plan and training.

Which is why I love the quote from Jade Teta when he said, "calories matter, I just don't count them."

You'll see in this example meal plan, and you'll get the full guide by clicking the link below to take the quiz – that calorie counting is not needed at all.

During the Metabolic Switch, you're not going to be <u>eating sugar, dairy, wheat, and gluten.</u>

One reason is we want to manage your powerful storage hormone, **insulin**.

It is the main hormone that regulates blood sugar levels and energy storage.

One of the functions of insulin is to tell fat cells to produce and store fat, along with holding on to the fat that they already carry.

So, insulin **stimulates lipogenesis (production of fat)** and **inhibits lipolysis (the burning of fat).**

It's also been shown a low-carb diet causes 2-3 times more weight loss compared to the standard low-fat diet (205, 206).

Another big benefit is that a high percentage of the fat lost on a low-carb diet comes from the belly area and the liver. This is the dangerous visceral fat that builds up in and around the organs, driving inflammation and disease (207, 208).

This is a graph from a study comparing low-carb and low-fat diets in overweight/obese women (209):

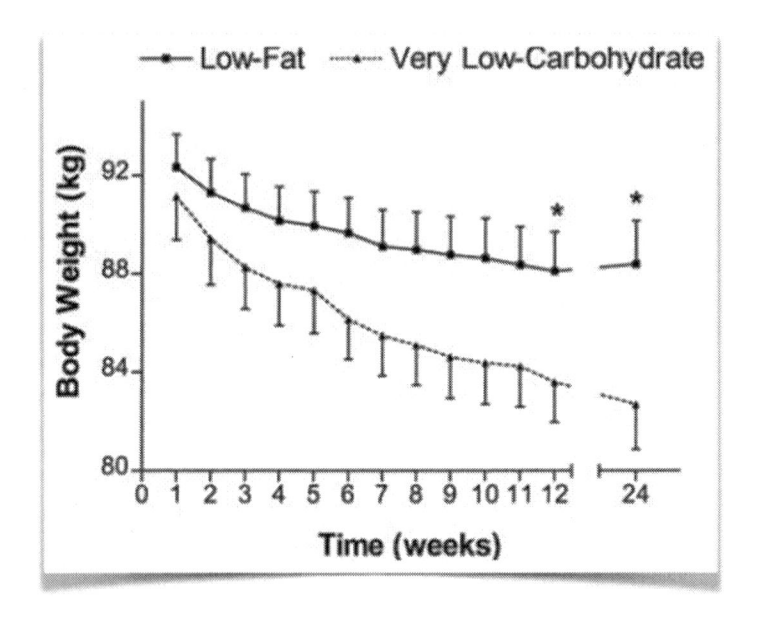

The low-carb group is eating until full, while the low-fat group is calorie restricted and hungry.

So by first having control of insulin by **choosing the right foods, we're able to "prime" your body to use fat for fuel.** This is because blood levels of the hormone insulin go way down when carb intake is reduced. High insulin levels contribute to fat storage, and low insulin levels facilitate fat burning.

Here is a graph from one study on low-carb diets (210):

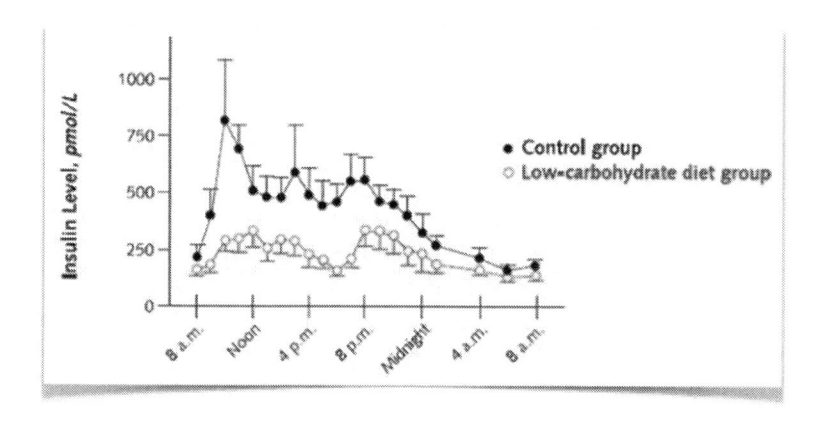

[Figure: Insulin Level (pmol/L) over time from 8 a.m. to 8 a.m., comparing Control group and Low-carbohydrate diet group]

Also, **let's be honest...**

Just taking the junk and processed foods out, is going to have a big benefit.

It is well known that increased food variety can drive increased calorie intake (211).

This is the where the processed foods are causing havoc in your body and brain. Causing you to be hungry from the chemical changes that these foods create.

Many of these foods are also highly rewarding, and the reward value of foods can impact how many calories we end up eating (212).

This is where your brain chemicals, one being dopamine, can make it harder for you to lose weight. As when you eat the processed foods that have a high reward, you're going to want more. And this is why relying on willpower doesn't work when trying to battle against a diet that isn't right for you.

On the flip side, starting with a Metabolic Priming Phase has a powerful effect on your appetite, helping you lose weight on 'autopilot' by having you feeling satisfied, and therefore, controlling the number of calories you eat.

Science shows that when people go low-carb, their appetite goes down, and they start eating fewer calories automatically (213).

In fact, studies that compare low-carb and low-fat diets usually restrict calories in the low-fat groups, while the low-carb groups are allowed to eat until they're full (214),

and this could be because of the effects on regulating hunger hormones such as leptin and ghrelin (215).

So, let's delve into the simple steps in your Metabolic Priming Phase.

And, let's cut straight to the chase…

You're not going to eat sugar, dairy, wheat, or gluten.

We've already covered some of the main reasons above as to why, as this is a simple step that takes out processed foods.

Quenching the Fire

Another reason why the 14-day Metabolic Priming Phase is so effective at kickstarting your fat loss and body transformation is through the lowering of inflammation.

You're probably familiar with the pain, swelling, redness, and heat that classically signify inflammation. It's something just about everyone out there has experienced.

Inflammation is part of the body's natural defense system. However, when your immune system shifts out of balance, inflammation can run rampant -- causing a chronic, smoldering fire inside your body that contributes to disease and weight gain.

The sugar you eat, high doses of the wrong oils and fats in your diet, hidden food allergens, lack of exercise, chronic stress, and hidden infections all trigger a raging, unseen inflammation deep in your cells and tissues.

Following the 14-Day Metabolic Switch will help you eliminate the excess swelling and fluid that accumulate in your tissues from food-induced chronic inflammation.

The problem is that chronic inflammation impairs the brain's ability to receive leptin's appetite suppressing message. The good news is that by eating foods to reduce inflammation, this will not only improve your heart health, it will improve your body's responsiveness to leptin. When that happens, you reduce inflammation, which makes it far easier to take off unwanted pounds.

During the initial 14-days, a lot of the weight you will lose will be from water. And you might (I have) hear people dismissively say, "Oh, you just lost water weight," they're right (at first), because eating foods you are allergic to causes inflammation, which leads to swelling and fluid retention.

Getting rid of this fluid by reducing inflammation is a GOOD thing, not a bad thing. It is what will allow your body to start the healing process, so you can achieve permanent weight loss and optimal health.

Breaking the Habit of You

Just 30 minutes ago, I got back from my morning walk and started listening to "Breaking The Habit Of Being Yourself" by Joe

Dispensa. I had to laugh out loud (by myself) when I sat down knowing that one of the biggest benefits of the 14-Day Metabolic Switch is that it helps you reset your eating and lifestyle habits.

And this is where I find so much of the 'secret sauce' lay in how our members have successfully lost weight and kept it off.

It's the step-by-step process that is easy to follow, and sets you up for the long-term success that is so important. This is why I covered in-depth in the previous Inner Game chapter why habits are such a critical part of your success.

It's by using the motivation that comes with your starting the 14-Day Metabolic Switch to get you moving in the direction. And then, having the path for you to easily follow that keeps you transforming into the body and person that you want to be.

What happens when we have become all motivated and decide "this is the time I'm getting in shape, and losing this weight!"

Getting in shape is playing carbs

Play one at a time

But, the truth is…

If I say don't think of a pink elephant…. you're thinking of a pink elephant.

So rather, let's focus on the abundant options you do have.

According to David Ludwig, MD, PhD, leading obesity researcher and professor of nutrition at Harvard University, our time and energy might be better spent paying more attention to what we eat rather than how much we eat. In fact, he goes on to say that our diet has the capacity to actually retrain our fat cells to burn more calories.

And this starts with…

STEP 1: Eat protein at each meal. Numerous studies show that protein can reduce appetite, boost metabolism, and help increase muscle mass, which is metabolically active and burns calories around the clock (216, 217).

This can range from grilled chicken to steak, to some hard-boiled eggs or even a scoop or two of protein in your green smoothie.

STEP 2: Eat an Abundant Amount of the "All You Can Eat Carbs." Focusing on the nutrient-dense, full of fiber vegetables is a key step.

It's probably the one main pieces of diet advice all nutritionists, gurus, and in between agree on… "eat more vegetables."

This is why we use the "All You Can Eat Carbs" list to give you a simple selection of foods that you can choose, and eat what you want.

Especially, leafy greens, which include kale, spinach, collards, and more…

Eating leafy greens is a great way to increase the volume of your meals without increasing the calories. Numerous studies show that meals and diets with a low energy density make people eat fewer calories overall (217).

Leafy greens are also incredibly nutritious and very high in all sorts of vitamins, minerals, and antioxidants. This includes calcium, which has been shown to aid fat burning in some studies. (218).

STEP 3: Add Healthy Fats. The Metabolic Switch is NOT about dramatically dropping your calories.

And where people go wrong is that they drop their fat intake along with taking away carbohydrates… turning it into a very low-calorie diet.

To avoid feeling flat, lethargic, or having high hunger that can turn into a binge-fest that can backfire on all your hard work… Focus on including fat in most meals.

Personally, I've tested a bunch of different foods and food combinations. And when it comes to fat, one of my favorite on the go sources is Phat Fudge. I talked about how Mary Shenouda "the paleo chef" helped me see and understand food in a way to better nourish ourselves.

Well, she is also the brilliant creator of Phat Fudge.

When it also comes to other good fats like coconut butter and nut butters, they can be easily overeaten. Where Phat Fudge is a neat one serving sachet that I always keep handy, so I never get "hangry."

We use the P-V-F-C Meal Model to know how to quickly put together each meal from a beginner to an advanced meal plan.

Protein	Veggies	Fats	Carbs
Chicken Breast	Cabbage	Coconut Oil	Sweet Potato
Turkey Breast	Broccoli	Olive Oil	Brown Rice
Beef	Spinach	Macadamia Nut Oil	Oats
Venison	Celery	Avocado	Quinoa
Lamb	Watercress	Nuts and Seeds	Beans
Kangaroo	Asparagus	Butter	Lentils
Salmon	Tomato		
White Fish	Zucchini		
Prawns	Cucumber		
Pork	Onion		
Whole Eggs	Snow Peas		
	Bok Choy		

Now a common question is, **"how many meals should I be eating?"**

There's a good chance you've heard, 'eat small meals more often to spike metabolism'… but the fact is, that's not true.

Most people I work with, along with myself, find around four meals a day works great.

Especially in the Metabolic Switch, I don't want you to think about how many meals you should be eating… Just eat when you're hungry, and stop when you're full.

This is why the main factor in this plan is your food choice.

In the example meal plan, I've included a smaller meal, including a shake, so you can quickly be on the go – as I know a big factor to make this work is that the meal plan fits into your lifestyle.

As the beauty of using the Metabolic Priming Phase is that the protein, good fats, and fibrous veg is going to have you feeling satisfied.

Step 4: Choose Your 'Eating Window.' Now it's time to start with an 8-hour window of when you are going to eat.

Is there any magic behind 8-hours…? NO!

From experience, we've found an 8-hour window is the easiest to start with, and then you can change it to what best suits you after the initial 14 days.

Let's say you choose to eat between 12pm and 8pm. You then have three easy steps to follow for the day:

#1: Have your first meal focused on a P-V-F meal.

Giving you a balanced blood sugar response with a strong injection of nutrition to have you thriving through the day.

Eat using the 80% principle. Which is to stop eating when you are 80% full. As it takes time for your stomach to communicate to your brain that you're satisfied, this gives you an easy bumper, so you don't overeat.

#2: Eat when you feel hungry.

Include meals in the My Body Diet.

#3: Enjoy your last meal at 8pm.

Now, there may be one question on your lips, and it could be…

"Chris, how many meals should I be eating in this eating window?"

It's a great question, as we squashed the myth of "eating every 2 hours to stoke your metabolism" in an earlier chapter. The Principle here is simple.

Eat a whole meal, and then eat another whole meal again when you get hungry. There is no need for snacking or grabbing a handful of food here and there. Simply enjoy your meal, and let your body digest and fuel yourself until you are ready to eat another meal.

The entire focus during the first 14-days is food quality and using each meal to be along the portion sizes that we've walked through before.

What's After the Metabolic Priming Phase?

This is designed to be your kickstart plan…

It goes for 14 days, as it gives your metabolism enough time to go through the 'switch' so you are burning fat for fuel effectively.

This isn't a 'diet' that you are meant to just keep following forever.

Most people will find a need to include carbohydrates back into their diet to further accelerate fat loss by helping hormonal balance and metabolism… But also, for the fact that you want to enjoy life and still eat your favorite foods.

This is why, in the next phase and onwards, we use a "smart carb approach." This is why improving your insulin sensitivity by starting with a metabolic switch phase is so important. Small bouts of low-carbohydrate eating can have a beneficial effect on our insulin sensitivity, so that when we do re-introduce carbohydrates later in the diet, we handle them more efficiently.

We start with carbohydrates that generally have a lower chance to be pro-inflammatory. So foods like sweet potato, pumpkin, and squash are common favorite options. This sticks with the idea that we are going for food quality and nutrient density. Rather than just wanting more "carbohydrate" in your diet.

And importantly, by following what I have for you in this book, you find what what's for YOU. So that you can get on enjoying your life and not be bogged down by trying to stick to a strict diet plan.

34

THE ONE COMMON FACTOR TO MAKING YOUR MEAL PLAN EASY.

There is a common factor that I continue to see being a common thread from the people I know that are highly successful in being able to lose weight and stay in shape. And once I started applying this, the penny finally dropped that one of the most important factors that will increase the likelihood of being able to stay in awesome shape is that it has to be simple and easy.

And that the lifestyle factor was a part of the equation that so many diets and weight loss programs didn't even consider. It wasn't until I first read The Four Hour Body, by Tim Ferriss, as he introduced the 'simple meal' idea.

The idea is that you want to have 2 to 3 meals that are your 'go to' choices throughout each day. This way, your shopping, cooking, preparing, cleaning, and entire meal preparation is fuss free and faster. Especially when starting, it's choosing the few meals that you enjoy eating, and ones that you are able to happily cook and prep so that it doesn't make life harder for you.

All too often, I hear that someone has bought a weight loss program; they open it up, and then are suddenly feeling like they are drowning in an ocean of information. When they peel themselves away from trying to read and understand everything, they get to the kitchen. Only to scratch their heads over how they now start shopping, prepping, cooking, and cleaning with all these new changes they are trying to follow.

The simple answer is that by eating simple meals with just a few whole foods, you can harness a powerful strategy for fat loss. This is Guenette's fundamental strategy for lowering the body fat set point (41).

This is where having your 2-4 "go-to" meals, that you cycle between, can become the staple of your meals throughout the week. Combining this with the 'easiest meal prep guide' I'm going to walk you through shortly, this is going to take away all the feelings of being overwhelmed.

It's the combination of the right food choices that normalizes the brain's sensitivity to the reward value of food, along with the minimizing the high variety of foods that can drive up the amount of food you eat (43). Then, on a lifestyle basis, this just makes life so much easier, and doesn't create the overwhelmed feeling and struggles that so many weight loss diets and recipe books create.

The biggest stumbling block for many is that the change in 'diet' comes along in a huge change, and brings confusion over what foods they need to eat, and where, when, and how they buy them. And then, when it comes to cooking and prepping meals each week, it all becomes too hard, and they revert back to their old ways.

This is why I've included a sample meal plan and also the recipe guide to give you everything you need to have a flying start. Plus, in the bonus download section (that you get free access to by having this book), there are even more meal plans, recipes, and videos walking you through the entire process.

This is a part of the secret sauce that allows you to get in shape, and not be feeling like you're constantly dieting or confused with how to make it 'fit' into your life.

Truthfully, I was forced to find out what works when it came to meal prep when I was prepping for my first fitness model competition. Now being a dad of two girls, my wife, Lauren, and I have four mouths and four tummies to nourish.

…and if you're like us, you don't have a lot of spare time to happily spend shopping, prepping, cooking, and cleaning.

So, let's get started.

I'm going to break this down into five easy steps, so you can go through each day and easily have your meals ready to go. Never getting caught out at work, traveling and coming home with nothing to eat.

We love meal prep because…

Meal prepping allows you to eat the foods you like, by easily getting ready all the foods, flavors, and recipes at once. You can make sure that each day, and at each meal, you're eating what you enjoy. So much of the time people are "falling off their diet" because they're stuck in situations where they can't choose the foods they want.

Meal prepping gives you super simple portion control, so you're not overeating.

By having everything ready to go and starting with the portion guide, you're not going to have meals where you have no idea of how much food is there. When you're busy and on the run, it's easy to overeat. This is where you can save yourself.

Meal prepping allows you to eat to the schedule that suits you.

It's not about eating to the clock. You should be filling yourself up with the foods by sitting down to eat when it suits you. We also love this because it stops us from eating at the computer or in front of the TV, and has us more aware of our foods.

Meal prepping saves you a lot of money each week.

When you're having to eat out all the time, it can be a real money pit. Save yourself a lot of cash by not having to choose to buy foods out all the time. Many members are always saying how much money they save during the work week by not having to go to cafes or local restaurants when at work.

Meal prepping save you from cheating

If you are eating out or grabbing food on the go, your food choices are far and few between. It's easy to get tempted when the choices are so limited.

We want to be able to combine the nutritional value of food

along with eating the right amount that suits your body and your goals.

In a way that fits in with your life and doesn't suck away your time, money and energy…

This is why, at My Body Blends, we combine the PVFC meal model (I'm going to show you all of this very soon) along with the portion control guide (yes, I'm even giving you this very soon) to have an easy jumpstart to eat the right foods and the right amounts.

For more advanced means, we can then move to tightening our focus to specific energy, hormonal, and macronutrient balance.

Before jumping into the guide, let's cover the importance of having the right food storage.

We want our stage to be BPA free, the right sizes to store for meals on the run or sit your big batch foods in the fridge, and they don't have crappy lids that don't snap together properly and can leak juices out later.

Lastly, before we jump into the five steps for meal prep, let's cover when you're going to do this.

For us, twice a week for the big batch is the easiest: Sundays and Wednesdays suit. If you're wondering whether there's a magic formula for this, NO.

Arlo isn't at school on Wednesdays, and Sundays we usually find after spending plenty of time in the sun and at the beach, it's nice to come back for a quick hour to get this all together before kicking back for the afternoon.

So, with the five steps of our meal prep guide, we break it down into;

The Most Important Macronutrient: Protein

We love our protein, as it helps preserve muscle when restricting energy intake for fat loss. A high-protein diet is more effective in reducing body fat and can include abdominal fat. Plus, protein keeps you fuller for longer, saving you from overeating.

The Three Flavor Tender Meats:

Spice it up to get all the health benefits, but also stop chewing on bland chicken or fish.

Using aluminum foil to divide your baking tray, chop your chicken and rub it down with your flavors of choice.

Vegetables

Don't be a salad dodger. You should love your veggies because they nourish you with a lot of what your body needs to thrive.

But it's ok… I hear people all the time not eating veggies just because they don't like the taste. So let's turn that around.

We break our veggie prep into; raw and cooked.

The Raw Veg Box

This is just a salad that I really enjoy and try to include.
Steamed or grilled

Starchy Carbs

There's no need to go into 101 different food combinations. The truth is, for you to have real success with getting in shape and having a super easy meal prep each week, you're going to only start with two (maybe three) options for each here.

Let's use rice and sweet potato (as that's what I'm making this week).

Cooking rice… Jeez. I hope I don't need to dive into this too much.

Seeing we live in Bali and are surrounded by rice paddies, we thought we would honor our environment and get some rice cooked. Throw it in with water, cook, then take out, pop it in the food box in the fridge.

For the sweet potato, it's simply going in the oven at the same time as the meats. This saves a lot of hassle, and everything is cooking at once.

Smoothie and Shakes

Bag up your smoothie ingredients so they are ready to go.

Quickly divide all your superfoods and ingredients so you can quickly throw them in the blender.

This is where I put together:
Protein Powder
Chia Seeds
Blueberries
Superfood Blend
Iced Greens

Quickly blend up your greens, and in the freezer, they go in an ice tray.

Then it's as simple as your iced greens and smoothie bags going in the blender at once.

There are also two other factors that we missed, but I did it on purpose because it's easy. This is;

Fruit:

The truth is, it's just throwing this alongside your meal, or having it in your bag or by your side for when you want.

Fats:

This is where you can drizzle your coconut/macadamia/olive oil over the top of your meals before you go, or have a small container full of nuts and seeds ready to go.

My favorite combo is: Brazil nuts, walnuts, macadamias, almonds, pepitas, and sunflower seeds. Or even adding a whole packet of Phat Fudge in.

35
THE KICKSTART WORKOUT GUIDE

Now it's time to walk through each of your workouts, and have full confidence that each second is designed to give you the biggest bang for your buck and the best results.

Firstly, we need to look at the key factors that make up your workouts, so you have the know-how to follow through with them whether they are at home, in a hotel room, or at a gym.

Exercise order:

Most workouts you've seen, and probably tried yourself, follow the rhythm of doing one exercise, resting, and repeating that one exercise for a few more sets. This is where we have a variety of changes to produce far superior results.

The letter/number combo that you find in your workout

programs refer to the exercise groups. So, you will perform all the sets of A exercises before starting into your B exercises, and so on.

For example, with the first workout below:

You will perform all the reps of the Deadlift, then move onto the Flat Chest Press. Rest for the time given (30 seconds), and then complete the next set until all sets given are complete. Then you move onto the B exercises.

Be sure to respect the rest period; 30 seconds is just enough time to switch exercise. The workout is purposely designed to pair the correct exercises together to get the best training effect.

Tempo (speed of movement with each exercise):

Tempo: Is a four-number sequence that dictates the speed you will perform each part of the movement.

We will use a squat as an example as I explain this to you.

The first number is the eccentric movement--when you lower the weight.

This will be you squatting down.

The second number is the point where you change the direction from lowering to lifting the weight.

This is when you are at the bottom of the squat. Any time given here is so you can keep tension in the muscle in the disadvantageous position, but not rest.

The third number is the concentric movement--when you lift the weight

This is when you are lifting yourself back up.

The fourth number is the point where you change direction from lifting to lowering the weight.

This is when you are at the top of the squat. Any time given here is for you to rest in the advantageous position, but not to lock your joints.

(A "0" indicates no time--simply move on to the next digit.)

Rest:

This is the time given before starting the next exercise. This is very important for Metabolic Resistance Training, as the training effect is designed to keep these rest periods short enough so that you get some rest. But long enough so that we can create the stimulus to get the best body transformation results.

Intensity:

It was in Halmstad, Sweden where I got a much-needed slap in the face.

I had just flown into Halmstad to immerse myself and learn from two of the world's best coaches, Charles Poliquin and Milos Sarcev. The internship was to learn the most effective techniques and coaching to transform bodies. Plus, we have the <u>pleasure</u> of training three times a day, as we all need to be able to experience what's going on to best coach it to others.

The very first workout was when it happened. I thought I was training hard, but it was a butterfly fart compared to what was expected of me now. And I am very, very thankful for that experience, as I attended many other internships, and searched out top coaches and athletes to train with to keep my own intensity of training high.

It's a fact, if you can have a world-class training program written for you but if you follow through with half-hearted effort and intensity, then your results will be lackluster. Though, if you follow through a mediocre program that still has basic principles of training adhered to, your results will be superior.

This is where being the coach and writing this, I can't stand by your side during your training sessions and get you to lift your intensity. This is where the responsibility (just like the rest of the guides I give you here ;)) lies squarely with you.

Choose a weight for your workouts that you can maintain great form, not break posture, and have only 1-2 reps left. Performing exercises to fail, especially as a beginner and with these multi-joint exercises, is not recommended in my experience. If you continue to progress and be true to yourself, then you will see fast and long-lasting results.

A1 - Deadlift 4 x 8 4010 30 seconds

A2 - Flat Bench. Neutral Grip DB Chest Press 4 x 12 3010 30 seconds

B1 - Front Foot Elevated Split Squat 4 x 12 (per leg) 2010 30 seconds

B2 - Neutral Grip Pulldown 4 x 15 3010 30 seconds

C1 - Leg Press or Squat 4 x 20 2010 30 seconds

C2 - Seated DB Shoulder Press with Neutral Grip 4 x 15 2010 30 seconds

Workout 2

A1 - DB Squats with Heels Elevated 4 x 15 3010 30 seconds

A2 - Bent Over BB Row 4 x 12 3010 30 seconds

B1 - Step Up 4 x 15 (per leg) 2010 30 seconds

B2 - Standing DB Shoulder Press 4 x 15 2010 30 seconds

C1 - Back Extension 4 x 15 2010 30 seconds

C2 - Push Up 4 x 15 2010 30 seconds

36
THE MY BODY DIET PROTOCOL

Has this happened to you?

You've been losing weight week to week, you're following your diet and your training plan, and it's going well.

The first few weeks, you can see you're progressing, and then, suddenly, the scale stops moving. Your weight loss stalls and you've hit a plateau. Now this can be frustrating; I've gone through this many times before.

And if you're sticking with your meal plan, your training hard, and not seeing the changes, it sucks, and it's disheartening.

There are a few different things you can do, which means you can jumpstart your body burning fat again. Now before we jump into those, there are two very important points we need to cover, and this is exactly what I do with my private clients and members.

Firstly, let's make sure you really have hit a weight loss plateau. Make sure you have been sticking with the plan. Before we go into changing the plan that you're currently using, if you're not sticking to the plan as needed – there's no point.

That's why, very soon in this chapter, I'll show you the importance of tracking what's really going on with your body.

But let's say you're eating four meals a day, which means you have 14 meals in a week. Now it's only three meals in a whole week to be off your plan for you to be missing your current weight loss by 10%.

So we can look at; is your meal plan to hard to follow, does it not suit your lifestyle so it's just a hard fit, is it too confusing, or what else can be an easy fix for you to easily go through each day and on plan.

Now thirdly, we need to look at what you're using to judge your progress. I am NOT a fan of using scale weight as the factor you are basing your body progressing with burning fat and building lean muscle.

<u>Scale weight is not telling you if you are burning fat,</u> holding more water, glycogen, or building some lean muscle, which all means the number you see really doesn't show you what your body is doing.

So I recommend you use girth measurements along with photos. Now with my members, they can update girth measurements and photos weekly in a cool custom software on their membership site, but for you, simply keeping the photos and writing down your girth measurements on the same day each week is an easy way to do it.

The big reason why I am giving this to you now is so that you have the know-how to be in charge of your body for the long-term. We start out with the 14-Day Metabolic Switch to give you the best start. Then we move onto increasing your food and carb intake until you get into the shape you want, and you find balance that has you looking, feeling, and performing the way you want each and every day.

So right now, let's walk through what you can do if, later on down the track, you hit a plateau (because you most certainly will).

So then if you have actually stopped progressing with fat loss, and you're sticking with your plan, we look at your training first.

For the majority of the time, I would rather start increasing someone's movement and exercise first, and then start dropping food.

And when it comes to increasing movement and exercise, we look at the foundation of training being your weight training. Simply, can you do an extra session per week? If not, cool, do we need to increase the volume or how much work you actually do in the workouts?

There are changes that could be changing the training split, so you can be training certain muscle groups more frequently, or do we use different parameters in the workouts, such as shorter rest intervals, lower to higher reps, or more.

Then we can look at cardio – and simply increasing it by a small amount (a great point I learned from John Meadows is there is no need to go from doing 20min of cardio to 60min of cardio per session because you hit a plateau). You're missing the huge benefits of the small amounts of stimulus needed for the body to progress in small increments in between.

So you could add an extra 10min training – now this could also mean you add a session of walking, or 10 minutes of Met Con if your energy levels are high and you are recovering well. For me, personally, I'd rather do more MRT workouts, and then increase the amount of walking I do. On the other hand, Lauren, my wife, enjoys doing more Met Con workouts.

There's no need to make it too complicated, do what you enjoy.

I know there are a lot of people jumping up and down about how you should only do HIIT (High-intensity Interval Training) style training for fat loss, and yes, it certainly has its merits, but if your physiological load is too high, your stressed out enough as it is, then adding that on top might not always be the best choice.

The trap so many people fall into is that they go into the "more is better" approach. And all of a sudden, they are training more than they should, and dramatically eating less food in the hope of chasing faster fat loss. This is not what the My Body Diet is about. This is about small, effective changes that put you in the driver's seat, and allows you to find balance for what best works for you.

Then we can decrease carbs – and I do because decreasing carbs will also drop your energy intake. And we can come to a better regulation of blood sugars and allow better fat lipolysis and oxidation to occur, meaning you're burning more fat.

Now when it comes to carbs, let's first make sure that you're choosing the right types of foods, but also, can we better time your carbs. Perhaps, you're better off putting your carbs around weight training, and in doing so, we may want to use a carb cycling method, or perhaps, a completely different change of stimulus is needed, such as using carb back loading, where you eat your day's carbs at the end of the day.

Now, start simple – a small reduction, at first, is all that's needed. I wanted to just mention a few more advanced methods to give you an idea of progression you can keep making. The biggest thing I don't want you to fall prey to is that thinking if a little is good, then a lot is better, so when taking carbs away, you take them all away.

Now I'm talking carbs and not protein and fats for a few reasons. For protein, we will stick to a number and it will be universal for you, not really changing. When it comes to fats as well, there is a threshold that we're not going to go under. Now depending when you start, we can determine whether you are a better fat burner, or sugar burner.

Or, whether you are more insulin sensitive or resistant, looking at how well you are at being efficient when eating carbs. As things like weight training are great for increasing insulin sensitivity, but also, the leaner you are, the better you will be, and also, other factors such as your metabolism and hormonal environment can get better as you progress through the program.

Now a great way to look at this is thanks to Dr. Jade Teta, I've had him on the podcast a few times and every one of those times is outstanding. A way I look at coaching people and myself is an eat less, move less scenario to also eat more, move more.

This is also why we start the My Body Diet with a "bottoms up" approach, kicking off with the 14-Day Metabolic Switch phase, and increasing food intake step-by-step. This helps build your metabolic capacity, as well as your body's ability to eat more food without gaining weight. So that when you do have times when your fat-loss plateaus, you are able to make the changes necessary.

I want to throw another point in here as well, and it's kind of two wrapped into one.

Firstly, we can look at refuel meals.

The idea of spiking your food and carbs is to help rebalance important hormones, such as thyroid and leptin, which can help jumpstart your body to burning fat again. There is also the method of a diet break – which is bringing your food up and have more rest, so more food and more rest for a short period.

If you've been dieting for quite some time, this is a method that has worked really well. And I've used it from mum and dads to top bikini competitors. One example is Kirsty when she was getting ready for a bikini and fitness model competition. Now for physique competitors, the technicalities of diet and training are much more dialed in, but she had hit a point where her body wasn't getting leaner, and I knew she was sticking to the plan.

Knowing what was going on with her body, I suggested a few days of eating more. Keeping the foods to great nutrient-dense choices, but really getting more carbs and fats in, and going with no training, lots of rest, meditation, extra sleep, and watching some funny movies.

After a couple of days, she then got back into the exact same plan as before, and that week, she had a massive drop. Especially, as we are all living busy lives, some down time to chill and relax is important. If your body is running on cortisol and adrenaline the whole time, there are nasty consequences.

So rather than looking at food and training, look at sleep and stress as well – can you get better quality or more sleep, and can you help your body chill out? It can be meditation, deep breathing, stretching, having a laugh, or going out for a surf.

You have to give yourself enough time to re-shape your body – weight loss isn't this plummeting straight line – you can't expect to be losing two to three pounds every week.

This was perfectly highlighted in a showcased interview with Ted Ryce. A world-class personal trainer that has coached the likes of Richard Branson to full-time mothers, and the two key aspects he highlights is consistency and trusting in the process.

After The 14-Day Metabolic Switch

They've been some of the most interesting and enjoyable conversations I've had.

Damon Hayhow is a coach and man I highly respect, and he has a track record that puts him as one of the leading voices in the field. Over time, I've interviewed and had the pleasure of talking with him; you can see the passion boil to the surface.

And it was the first time we talked, immediately after hanging up on our call, that I looked down to my notes (that I could barely read, as I was writing so quickly), that I decided to change the entire coaching process I had set up for our members.

As he brings to the forefront and reminds us of one of the most important factors that matter for when it comes to you being able to get to the body and health you want.

And that is: Is what you are doing…

<u>Is it working?</u>

Are you measuring your results on a consistent basis so that you are confident in what you are doing is working or not?

As one of the biggest traps I see so many people fall into is that they are clueless as to what is working for them.

This entire book is NOT to give you an exact meal plan or weight loss program to follow for the rest of your life. This is to highlight the key principles, give you the best starting block, and to empower you to be in charge of your own body and health.

And you cannot do that if you are not taking note of how your body and day by day performances are progressing.

To give you a clear path to follow, let me share with you what we do with our members and private clients.

Each Friday, the members log into their account on our site, and they have a simple to use progress tracker. Simply being able to upload a front photo, girth measurement, and weight (which is all kept private to themselves), and the nifty piece of custom software we have developed for our members then shows their progress.

You can take this exact formula and copy it without being a member. Simply choose a day of the week that you will take your updates on, and decide on what you are going to track. Ultimately, testing body fat with a DEXA scan is ideal, but it's not realistic for me to expect our members to do that. So by using the three measurements, we can have a clear idea of how your body is progressing.

But there is a bigger reason why I do this for you...

One of the flaws that we can have that constantly has us frustrated is seeing the gap between where we are now, and where we want to go.

This gap becomes a constant void and stressor because it feels like we are chasing after something, and all the hard work and effort we are putting in... Is not staying off.

But that's not how we should be looking at it. Progress is never in the future. Progress is in the past.

We need to look backward to see where we have come from.

So by measuring backward, we are now able to see the fantastic progress that we are making.

By comparing what our body or health markers are now to a month ago, we can see that we have made leaps and gains.

This might sound like semantics to start with, but it's the switch that helps your brain appreciate what you are doing, and what you are achieving.

I've had countless clients sit down in front of me or get calls from them, all depressed. They thought that they haven't been progressing because they saw a glimpse of themselves passing a mirror, or they just feel "off." But when we look at the actual measurements, all of sudden, they perk up, feel great, and realize that they are making great progress.

For the easiest steps to tracking your progress -

1. Choose one objective outcome-based measurement that you are going to track (Example: Your waist measurement).
2. Choose a daily process focused measurement that you are going to track (Example: Following your plan for each meal of the day).
3. Choose a day of the week at the same time, where you look back and compare your results.
4. Decide on what changes need to happen moving forward.
5. Celebrate your wins!

Now, you can certainly choose more measurements to track, and with the surge of 'biohacking' enthusiast and self-quantification becoming all the rage from body fat to sleep tracking, to Heart Rate Variability training and beyond, the amount of tracking and self-quantification can start to become a hindrance rather than a positive. So I always rather start small, and build-up, if needed.

If you start with the smallest and easiest steps, it will give you the best possibility of following through, and actually creating the habits and behaviors that set you up for long-term success. Again, this swings around into why I have designed the My Body Diet and the programs the way I have; so that you have the highest chance of success.

37
THE MY BODY FOR LIFE

I'm sorry…

I LIED to you.

This book was wrapped with the design to have you lose weight faster than you ever have before, easier than you ever thought possible. And have you easily keep it off.

But that's not why I wrote this for you.

You getting into great shape, is a side effect.

Everything that I have laid out here for you is with the design of putting your health first.

Firstly, to have your body not just surviving our modern-day lives (and with the hope to dodge the bullets that are our main killers being cancer and heart disease are), it's to have you thriving. With boundless energy for you to be who you want to be.

Secondly, it's so that you are performing day in, day out, with your brain firing on all cylinders. So you are not only fueling your brain to be performing at its best, but also, so that you're not getting caught up in the petty thoughts and behaviors that can lower your energy and capabilities that can happen when you are undernourished and over stressed.

As for myself, I want to be able to thrive each day.

I want to be the best husband and lover I can be. To have the sexual vigor of a twenty-year-old. Not a guy losing my 'manliness' because I can't get an erection to satisfy my wife. Not a guy that is so caught up with my own 'stuff,' that I lose focus on the importance of the little things that really matter. I want to have the spontaneity and drive that has my wife feeling like a queen.

I want to be the best father who can not only protect and provide for my family, but have the energy where I can run and goof around with them at all hours of the day. I don't want to sloth on the couch with "daddy's too tired" or hurt my back throwing my girls around in the pool. I want to be the best example I can be for them to grow into the world-changing, loving humans they deserve to be.

I want to be the best entrepreneur, so I have the creativity, discipline, and power to bring to life the value, products, information, and help that changes millions lives all around the world. I don't want to be hitting a wall mid-afternoon and being low on energy, which only sucks away from the success that I see is achieved by how great of an impact I can make. I want to have the physical and mental prowess that empowers the companies I run to leave a positive footprint.

I want to be the best version of myself. And if you want that for yourself, then join me and the community, so we can do it together.

It was having dinner with Katrina Ruth, which I'm very proud to say is my partner with My Body Blends, that sparked a massive change. We had begun a bit of a ritual that whenever we were in the same city, we would get together for dinner, catch up, and 'solve the problems of the world.' Though this time, our conversation turned to why "compromise" is such a dirty word.

Why is it that, as a society, we can so easily fall into living a life full of compromises? Why is it so accepted that we can use the excuse of "I'm busy with work," "I have kids," or the plethora of other pathetic excuses that, truthfully, are only a self-limiting belief that is put upon ourselves by saying it?

> **Shelly Somerville** 7:19am
> Yes!! That's what I'm after
> Thank you! I'd really appreciate that.
>
> You have changed my life, I never thought I would be eating this well and actually enjoying it. And not to mention the body transformation in such a short time.

> **Katie Wearmouth**
> 1 hr
>
> Just reflecting back on the last 6 months and how far I have come. It hasn't been an easy year but I chose to turn that around and focus on my health and fitness before anything else. I couldn't be happier and now I have Chris Dufey in my corner, I know I can achieve anything I set out to do. This is only the beginning of something bigger and better.

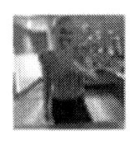

You can have it all.

You can have the body.

You can have the financial success.

You can have the relationships.

You can have the health.

You can have the happiness.

You can have successful life; however you want to define it.

And that is why this book has been written, so you become the best version of yourself.

And this is why I want you to join myself and the My Body Blends community to become a part of the movement that is for men and women taking charge of our health, being in great shape, and being able to live the lives that we want to.

Life is too short to be stressing over how many calories you're eating if you're training is right for you, or why you're stuck not being able to lose weight.

I don't want you to take your last breathes having regret. Not being the person you want to be, not achieving what you wanted. All because your body, confidence, health, or self-belief was holding you back.

The traditional diets want you to believe that you are broken. Because then, they can sell you something that will always have you chasing after something you can't attain. Just like the carrot at the end of the stick. And that's how they can make money from you for the rest of your life.

The fact is though.

You can upgrade your life.

You can become the best version of yourself and "have it all."

And we believe it starts by transforming your body and your brain.

I'm looking forward to having you join us, and seeing your transformation and results.

Thank you!

REFERENCES

1. http://jcem.endojournals.org/content/89/6/2963.short
2. http://www.ncbi.nlm.nih.gov/pmc/articles/PMC2673878/
3. http://www.ncbi.nlm.nih.gov/pubmed/23140226
4. http://www.ncbi.nlm.nih.gov/pubmed/12174324
5. http://www.ncbi.nlm.nih.gov/pubmed/20565999
6. http://www.ncbi.nlm.nih.gov/pubmed/11838888
7. http://www.ncbi.nlm.nih.gov/pubmed/18469147
8. http://www.ncbi.nlm.nih.gov/pubmed/15466943
9. http://www.ncbi.nlm.nih.gov/pubmed/10375057
10. http://www.ncbi.nlm.nih.gov/pubmed/19153580
11. http://annals.org/article.aspx?articleid=717451
12. http://www.nature.com/nrendo/journal/v2/n8/abs/ncpendmet0220.html
13. http://atvb.ahajournals.org/content/25/12/2451.full
14. http://www.ncbi.nlm.nih.gov/pubmed/8532024
15. http://www.nature.com/ijo/journal/v14/n10/pdf/0802753a.pdf
16. http://onlinelibrary.wiley.com/doi/10.1111/j.1432-1033.1989.tb14842.x/pdf
17. https://www.ncbi.nlm.nih.gov/pubmed/10797147
18. https://www.ncbi.nlm.nih.gov/pmc/articles/PMC4018593/
19. https://www.sciencedaily.com/releases/2016/11/161129091143.htm
20. http://www.sciencemag.org/cgi/content/abstract/sci;314/5975/214

21. https://clinicaltrials.gov/ct2/show/study/NCT02530385
22. http://mayoclinicproceedings.com/content/83/4/460.full#_jmp0_
23. http://www.ajcn.org/cgi/content/abstract/87/3/534
24. http://www.cell.com/cell/abstract/S0092-8674(15)01481-6
25. http://www.ncbi.nlm.nih.gov/pubmed/22492122
26. https://examine.com/nutrition/do-i-need-to-eat-six-times-a-day-to-keep-my-metabolism-high/#ref1
27. http://www.ncbi.nlm.nih.gov/pubmed/11497044
14. http://www.ncbi.nlm.nih.gov/pubmed/17214046
29. http://www.sciencedirect.com/science/article/pii/S000142230501151X
30. http://www.ncbi.nlm.nih.gov/pubmed/12144716
31. https://www.ncbi.nlm.nih.gov/pubmed/17723014
32. https://www.ncbi.nlm.nih.gov/pubmed/5010404
33. Kent C. Berridge, "The Debate over Dopamine's Role in Reward: The Case for Incentive Salience," Psychopharmacology 191, no. 3 (2007): 391-431.
34. Xiao Tian Wang and Robert D. Dvorak, "Sweet Future: Fluctuating Blood Glucose Levels Affect Future Discounting," Psychological Science 21 no. 2 (2010): 183-88. doi: 10.1177/ 0956797609358096.
35. Thomas L. Kash, William P. Nobis, Robert T. Matthews, and Danny G. Winder, "Dopamine Enhances Fast Excitatory Synaptic Transmission in the Extended Amygdala by a CRF-R1-Dependent Process," Journal of Neuroscience 14, no. 51 (2008): 13856-65. doi: 10.1523/ JNEUROSCI. 4715-08.2008.
36. http://articles.mercola.com/sites/articles/archive/2015/09/07/nutritional-value-beats-calorie-count.aspx#_edn2
37. https://www.ncbi.nlm.nih.gov/pubmed/11882927
38. http://www.apa.org/pubs/journals/releases/xlm-a0036577.pdf
39. Christian Frøsig and Erik A. Richter, "Improved Insulin Sensitivity after

Exercise: Focus on Insulin Signaling," Obesity 17, no. S3: S15-S20. doi: 10.1038/ oby. 2009.383; John J. Dubé, Katelyn Fleishman, Valentin Rousson, Bret H. Goodpaster, and Francesca Amati, "Exercise Dose and Insulin Sensitivity: Relevance for Diabetes Prevention," Medicine and Science of Sports and Exercise 44, no. 5 (2012): 793-9. doi: 10.1249/ MSS. 0b013e31823f679f.

40. Angelo Tremblay, Jean-Aimé Simoneau, and Claude Bouchard, "Impact of Exercise Intensity on Body Fatness and Skeletal Muscle Metabolism," Metabolism 43, no. 7 (1994): 814-18. doi: 10.1016/ 0026-0495(94) 90259-3; Jeffrey W. King, "A Comparison of the Effects of Interval Training vs. Continuous Training on Weight Loss and Body Composition in Obese Pre-Menopausal Women" (Thesis, East Tennessee State University, 2001), http:// static.ow.ly/ docs/ Interval Training v Continuous Training_5gS.pdf; Margarita S. Treuth, Gary R. Hunter, and Michael Williams, "Effects of Exercise Intensity on 24-h Energy Expenditure Expenditure and Substrate Oxidation," Medicine and Science of Sports and Exercise 14, no. 9 (1996): 1138-43; E. Gail Trapp, Donald J. Chisholm, Judith Freund, and Stephen H. Boutcher, "The Effects of High-Intensity Intermittent Exercise Training on Fat Loss and Fasting Insulin Levels of Young Women," International Journal of Obesity 32, no. 4 (2008): 684-691. doi: 10.1038/ sj.ijo. 0803781.

41. Bryant, Cedric X. 101 Frequently Asked Questions about "Health & Fitness" and "Nutrition & Weight Control". Sagamore Publishing, 1999

42. Guyenet, S. (2012, August 29). Obesity; Old solutions for a new problem. 2011 Ancestral Health Symposium UCLA. Retrieved from https:// www.youtube.com/ watch? v = srqFz0fO8xk.

43. Cabanac, M., & Rabe, E. F. (1976). Influence of a monotonous food on body weight regulation in humans. Physiol Behav. 17(4), 675-8

44. http://www.sciencedirect.com/science/article/pii/S1751499110000545

45. http://journals.plos.org/plosone/article?id=10.1371/journal.pone.0038632

46. Bellisle F, McDevitt R, Prentice AM Meal frequency and energy balance. Br J Nutr. (1997)

47. Webber J, Macdonald IA The cardiovascular, metabolic and hormonal changes accompanying acute starvation in men and women. Br J Nutr. (1994)

48. Heilbronn LK, et al Alternate-day fasting in non-obese subjects: effects on body weight, body composition, and energy metabolism. Am J Clin Nutr. (2005)

49. http://ajcn.nutrition.org/content/early/2014/06/04/ajcn.114.089573.abstract

50. http://jn.nutrition.org/content/137/11/2539S.full

51. http://www.ncbi.nlm.nih.gov/pubmed/12583961

52. http://www.ncbi.nlm.nih.gov/pubmed/17183309

53. http://care.diabetesjournals.org/content/33/10/2277.full

54. http://www.ncbi.nlm.nih.gov/pubmed/15894105

55. http://onlinelibrary.wiley.com/doi/10.1111/j.1365-2982.2010.01664.x/full

56. http://www.ncbi.nlm.nih.gov/pubmed/22555633

57. http://www.ncbi.nlm.nih.gov/pubmed/16918875

58. http://www.ncbi.nlm.nih.gov/pubmed/21050146

59. http://www.ncbi.nlm.nih.gov/pubmed/12490960

60. http://www.ncbi.nlm.nih.gov/pubmed/12490959

61. http://www.jci.org/articles/view/57132

62. http://www.ncbi.nlm.nih.gov/pmc/articles/PMC3248304/

63. http://www.ncbi.nlm.nih.gov/pmc/articles/PMC3319208/

64. http://www.ncbi.nlm.nih.gov/pubmed/21050146

65. http://jn.nutrition.org/content/130/2/272S.full

66. http://www.ncbi.nlm.nih.gov/pubmed/17091430

67. http://www.ncbi.nlm.nih.gov/pubmed/21676152
68. http://www.ncbi.nlm.nih.gov/pmc/articles/PMC3856431/
69. http://www.ncbi.nlm.nih.gov/pmc/articles/PMC4258944/
70. http://www.ncbi.nlm.nih.gov/pubmed/25926512
71. http://www.ncbi.nlm.nih.gov/pmc/articles/PMC4424378/
72. http://www.ncbi.nlm.nih.gov/pubmed/16400055/
73. http://www.sciencedirect.com/science/article/pii/S1550413106002713
74. http://press.endocrine.org/doi/abs/10.1210/jc.2009-0949
75. http://www.ncbi.nlm.nih.gov/pubmed/22188045
76. http://www.ncbi.nlm.nih.gov/pubmed/16469977
77. http://www.ncbi.nlm.nih.gov/pmc/articles/PMC524030/
78. http://ajcn.nutrition.org/content/101/3/496.abstract
79. http://www.ncbi.nlm.nih.gov/pubmed/8856395
80. http://www.ncbi.nlm.nih.gov/pmc/articles/PMC4258944/
81. https://www.ncbi.nlm.nih.gov/pubmed/20847729
82. http://www.nutritionj.com/content/13/1/80
83. http://www.ncbi.nlm.nih.gov/pubmed/15303109
84. http://www.ncbi.nlm.nih.gov/pubmed/15466943
85. http://www.ncbi.nlm.nih.gov/pubmed/22935440
86. http://onlinelibrary.wiley.com/doi/10.1046/j.1467-789x.2000.00019.x/full
87. http://www.ncbi.nlm.nih.gov/pubmed/14710168
88. Jenkins, A.B., et al., Carbohydrate intake and short-term regulation of leptin in humans. Diabetologia, 1997. 40(3): p. 348-51.
89. Mars M, Graaf C, Groot CP, van Rossum CT, Kok FJ. Fasting leptin and appetite responses induced by a 4-day 65%-energy-restricted diet. Int J Obes (Lond). 2006 Jan;30(1):122-8.
90. Keim, N.L., J.S. Stern, and P.J. Havel, Relation between circulating leptin

concentrations and appetite during a prolonged, moderate energy deficit in women. Am J Clin Nutr, 1998. 68(4): p. 794-801.

91. http://www.jstor.org/discover/10.1086/663212?uid=3739776&uid=2&uid=4&uid=3739256&sid=21102001683777

92. Schoeller DA. The energy balance equation: looking back and looking forward are two very different views. Nutr Rev. 2009;67(5):249–254. doi:10.1111/j.1753-4887.2009.00197.x

93. Buchholz AC, Schoeller DA. Is a calorie a calorie? Am J Clin Nutr. 2004;79(5):899S–906S. Available at: http://eutils.ncbi.nlm.nih.gov/entrez/eutils/elink.fcgi?dbfrom=pubmed&id=15113737&retmode=ref&cmd=prlinks.

94. Ello-Martin JA, Ledikwe JH, Rolls BJ. The influence of food portion size and energy density on energy intake: implications for weight management. Am J Clin Nutr. 2005;82(1 Suppl):236S–241S. Available at: http://ajcn.nutrition.org/content/82/1/236S.long.

95. Rolls BJ, Morris EL, Roe LS. Portion size of food affects energy intake in normal-weight and overweight men and women. Am J Clin Nutr. 2002;76(6):1207–1213. Available at: http://ajcn.nutrition.org/content/76/6/1207.long.

96. http://www.eurekalert.org/pub_releases/2015-03/tes-l3m030515.php

97. http://www.ajcn.org/content/93/6/1229.abstract?sid=ee6e80cd-d844-4103-ade3-82d9b41b9357

98. http://annals.org/article.aspx?articleid=1379773

99. https://www.ncbi.nlm.nih.gov/pubmed/24965304

100. https://www.ncbi.nlm.nih.gov/pubmed/24524148

101. https://www.ncbi.nlm.nih.gov/pubmed/24433933

102. https://www.ncbi.nlm.nih.gov/pubmed/24848969

103. https://www.ncbi.nlm.nih.gov/pubmed/24458353
104. https://www.ncbi.nlm.nih.gov/pubmed/24367384
105. http://www.ncbi.nlm.nih.gov/pubmed/9467584
106. http://www.ncbi.nlm.nih.gov/pubmed/9467584
107. http://www.ncbi.nlm.nih.gov/pubmed/7673425
108. http://www.ncbi.nlm.nih.gov/pubmed/9467584
109. http://www.ncbi.nlm.nih.gov/pubmed/20604869
110. http://www.pnas.org/content/100/20/11696.abstract
111. http://www.psychosomaticmedicine.org/content/65/4/564.short
112. http://psycnet.apa.org/psycinfo/2008-14857-004
113. http://link.springer.com/article/10.1023/B:COTR.0000045557.15923.96
114. http://online.liebertpub.com/doi/abs/10.1089/acm.2006.12.817
115. http://ajp.psychiatryonline.org/article.aspx?articleID=168746
116. http://psycnet.apa.org/journals/str/12/2/164/
117. http://www.psychosomaticmedicine.org/content/62/5/613.short
118. http://www.psychosomaticmedicine.org/content/65/4/564.short
119. http://www.sciencedirect.com/science/article/pii/S0889159112004758
120. http://www.sciencedirect.com/science/article/pii/S0889159112001894%2020
121. http://www.sciencedirect.com/science/article/pii/S1053810010000681
122. http://link.springer.com/article/10.3758/CABN.7.2.109#page-1
123. http://dl.acm.org/citation.cfm?id=1979862
124. Hill AM, Buckley JD, Murphy KJ, Howe PR. Combining fish-oil supplements with regular aerobic exercise improves body composition and cardiovascular disease risk factors. Am J Clin Nutr. 2007 May;85(5):1267-74.
125. Smith, G. Et al. Omega-3 Polyunsaturated Fatty Acids Augment the muscle protein anabolic response to hyper aminoacidemia- hyperinsulinemia in

healthy young and middle-aged men and women. Clinical Sciences. 2011. 121(6), 267-278

126. http://www.ncbi.nlm.nih.gov/pubmed/12438303

127. http://www.ncbi.nlm.nih.gov/pubmed/10617969

114. http://www.ncbi.nlm.nih.gov/pubmed/20500789/

129. http://www.ncbi.nlm.nih.gov/pmc/articles/PMC3279313/

130. http://jama.jamanetwork.com/article.aspx?articleid=195646

131. http://www.ncbi.nlm.nih.gov/pubmed/24026545

132. http://www.ncbi.nlm.nih.gov/pubmed/16741195

133. http://www.ncbi.nlm.nih.gov/pubmed/18789910

134. http://www.ncbi.nlm.nih.gov/pubmed/22254005

135. http://www.ncbi.nlm.nih.gov/pubmed/26571503

136. http://www.ncbi.nlm.nih.gov/pubmed/21501117

137. http://www.ncbi.nlm.nih.gov/pubmed/26571503

138. http://www.ncbi.nlm.nih.gov/pubmed/15481762

139. http://www.ncbi.nlm.nih.gov/pubmed/?term=chlorella+kyoto+Japan+2008

140. http://www.ncbi.nlm.nih.gov/pubmed/19723054

141. http://www.ncbi.nlm.nih.gov/pubmed/24333277

142. Li Y, Wang C, Zhu K, Feng RN, Sun CH. Effects of multivitamin and mineral supplementation on adiposity, energy expenditure and lipid profiles in obese Chinese women. Int J Obes (Lond). 2010 Jun;34(6):1070-7.

143. http://www.cnn.com/2014/12/31/health/magnesium-deficiency-health/index.html

144. http://www.ncbi.nlm.nih.gov/pubmed/6299329

145. http://pmid.us/11595455

146. http://www.ncbi.nlm.nih.gov/pubmed/17519496

147. http://pmid.us/4018443

148. http://pmid.us/11595455

149. http://www.ncbi.nlm.nih.gov/pubmed/19761418

150. http://www.organic-center.org/reportfiles/Oregon_Tilth_2008%20%5BCompatibility%20Mode%5D.pdf

151. http://www.berkeley.edu/news/media/releases/99legacy/5-18-1999.html

152. http://www.ncbi.nlm.nih.gov/pubmed/18309763?dopt=AbstractPlus

153. http://lpi.oregonstate.edu/mic/minerals/copper

154. http://www.ncbi.nlm.nih.gov/pmc/articles/PMC1495189/

155. http://www.ncbi.nlm.nih.gov/pubmed/9721056?dopt=AbstractPlus

156. http://www.ajcn.org/content/71/3/682.long

157. http://www.ana-jana.org/Journal/journals/ACF5FB7.pdf

158. http://pubs.acs.org/doi/abs/10.1021/jf020635c

159. http://www.ipni.net/ppiweb/bcrops.nsf/$webindex/70ABDB50A75463F085257394001B157F/$file/07-4p12.pdf

160. https://www.ncbi.nlm.nih.gov/pubmed/16323755

161. http://www.ewg.org/reports/farmedPCBs/

162. http://www.ajcn.org/content/89/5/1543S.abstract

163. http://www.ncbi.nlm.nih.gov/pubmed/15614200

164. http://www.ncbi.nlm.nih.gov/pubmed/16320857

165. http://www.ncbi.nlm.nih.gov/pubmed/18841408

166. http://www.crnusa.org/CRNfoundation/HCCS/

167. http://www.ncbi.nlm.nih.gov/pubmed/17556681

168. http://jn.nutrition.org/content/133/1/249S.full.pdf+html

169. https://www.ncbi.nlm.nih.gov/pubmed/24912386

170. http://www.sciencedirect.com/science/article/pii/S0091467412001043

171. https://www.ncbi.nlm.nih.gov/pubmed/19007054

172. https://www.ncbi.nlm.nih.gov/pubmed/25511750
173. https://www.ncbi.nlm.nih.gov/pubmed/18684338/
174. https://www.ncbi.nlm.nih.gov/pubmed/25884980
175. https://www.ncbi.nlm.nih.gov/pubmed/14001147
176. http://www.sciencedirect.com/science/article/pii/S1756464612001399
177. https://www.ncbi.nlm.nih.gov/pubmed/23614897
178. https://www.ncbi.nlm.nih.gov/pubmed/24299712
179. https://www.ncbi.nlm.nih.gov/pubmed/23614897
180. http://www.sciencedirect.com/science/article/pii/S235293931600004X
181. https://www.ncbi.nlm.nih.gov/pubmed/27413138
182. https://www.ncbi.nlm.nih.gov/pubmed/25879690
183. https://www.ncbi.nlm.nih.gov/pubmed/19338686
184. https://www.ncbi.nlm.nih.gov/pubmed/25862297
185. https://www.ncbi.nlm.nih.gov/pubmed/27509521
186. https://www.ncbi.nlm.nih.gov/pubmed/26706022
187. https://www.ncbi.nlm.nih.gov/pubmed/17311983
188. http://www.ncbi.nlm.nih.gov/pubmed/17183309
189. http://www.ncbi.nlm.nih.gov/pubmed/19043404/
190. http://www.ncbi.nlm.nih.gov/pubmed/19640952
191. http://www.ncbi.nlm.nih.gov/pubmed/16400055/
192. http://www.ncbi.nlm.nih.gov/pubmed/16400055/
193. http://www.ncbi.nlm.nih.gov/pubmed/16950139
194. http://www.ncbi.nlm.nih.gov/pubmed/22188045
195. http://www.ncbi.nlm.nih.gov/pmc/articles/PMC524030/
196. http://www.ncbi.nlm.nih.gov/pubmed/8862477
197. http://www.ncbi.nlm.nih.gov/pubmed/25033958
198. http://www.sciencedirect.com/science/article/pii/S1057740814000291

199. http://www.ncbi.nlm.nih.gov/pmc/articles/PMC1431986/
200. http://www.cscb.northwestern.edu/jcpdfs/frank01.pdf
201. http://www.sleepfoundation.org/article/how-sleep-works/how-much-sleep-do-we-really-need
202. http://www.ncbi.nlm.nih.gov/pubmed/22691622
203. https://www.ncbi.nlm.nih.gov/pmc/articles/PMC4209489/
204. https://www.nytimes.com/2016/09/13/well/eat/how-the-sugar-industry-shifted-blame-to-fat.html
205. http://onlinelibrary.wiley.com/doi/10.1111/j.1464-5491.2007.02290.x/full
206. http://www.nejm.org/doi/full/10.1056/NEJMoa022637
207. http://www.nutritionandmetabolism.com/content/1/1/13
208. http://www.ncbi.nlm.nih.gov/pubmed/21367948
209. http://www.ncbi.nlm.nih.gov/pubmed/12679447
210. http://annals.org/article.aspx?articleid=718265
211. http://www.ncbi.nlm.nih.gov/pubmed/11393299
212. http://www.ncbi.nlm.nih.gov/pmc/articles/PMC3319208/
213. http://www.ncbi.nlm.nih.gov/pubmed/17214046
214. http://press.endocrine.org/doi/full/10.1210/jc.2002-021480
215. http://www.nature.com/ejcn/journal/v67/n7/full/ejcn201390a.html
216. http://www.ncbi.nlm.nih.gov/pubmed/15466943
217. http://www.ncbi.nlm.nih.gov/pubmed/8862477
218. http://www.ncbi.nlm.nih.gov/pubmed/17556681
219. http://www.ncbi.nlm.nih.gov/pmc/articles/PMC3786545/
220. http://www.ncbi.nlm.nih.gov/pmc/articles/PMC1431986/

AUTHOR'S NOTE

Thank you so much for getting your copy of Craving The Truth.

I would love to hear from you. Tell me what you enjoyed and what you used from the book.

Please take a photo and tag me on social media. I love connecting and I'll answer as many of your questions as I can.

I wrote this book largely for myself and to empower my friends, family and community. And then it changed my life. I certainly hope it does the same for you.

I wish you the best of luck. Carve your own path.

All the best,

Chris Dufey

My website:
http://cravingthetruth.com/

I'm @chrisdufey on all the major social media platforms.

Manufactured by Amazon.ca
Bolton, ON